Step by Step
Reading Pentacam
Topography

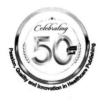

Notification

The information provided via this book is intended to build systematic skills and to assist in decision making. However, it is still the surgeon's full responsibility to make the decision based on clinical examination and full investigations. Surgeons must arrive at their own independent determination regarding the proper treatment for their patients and are solely responsible for the refractive outcome. Therefore, the author accepts no liability whatsoever for any direct or consequential loss arising from any use of the information contained in this book.

Step by Step®
Reading Pentacam Topography

(Basics and Clinical Applications)

Third Edition

Mazen M Sinjab
MD MSc ABOphth PhD FRCOphth (Hons) CertLRS (London)
Professor of Ophthalmology, Damascus University, Syria
Visiting Professor, Hassan II University, Casablanca, Morocco
Consultant Ophthalmic Surgeon
Phaco-Refractive Surgeon
Dr Mazen Sinjab Eye Clinic, Dubai, UAE
Al Zahra Eye Center, Damascus, Syria

JP
medical
publishers

London • New Delhi

Headquarters
Jaypee Brothers Medical Publishers (P) Ltd
4838/24, Ansari Road, Daryaganj
New Delhi 110 002, India
Phone: +91-11-43574357
Fax: +91-11-43574314
Email: jaypee@jaypeebrothers.com

Overseas Office
J.P. Medical Ltd
83 Victoria Street, London
SW1H 0HW (UK)
Phone: +44 20 3170 8910
Fax: +44 (0)20 3008 6180
Email: info@jpmedpub.com

Website: www.jaypeebrothers.com
Website: www.jaypeedigital.com

Step by Step® Reading Pentacam Topography (Basics and Clinical Applications)

First Edition: 2010
Second Edition: 2015
Third Edition: **2021**

ISBN: 978-1-78779-129-9

Printed at: Samrat Offset Pvt. Ltd.

Dedicated to

My dear Father Mohamad (may God rest his soul),
who implanted in my soul the love of excellence
I will mention his name with my name all my life

My Mother Almasah (may God rest her soul),
who implanted in my heart the love of the
poor and helping others

My Wife Ruba (may God save her),
For the unwavering support in every detail in my life

My students and followers
whose comments, suggestions, and corrections
were critical for all my books

I dedicate this book
Mazen Mohamad Sinjab

Preface to the Third Edition

This is the Third edition of *Step By Step Reading Corneal Topography*.

Reading corneal tomography is a science and an art. By reading systematically, a sense develops to distinguish what is normal from what is abnormal.

With the advancement in tomographic devices and the newly added features, corneal tomography became a keystone in the workup of all types of refractive surgery and modern cataract surgery.

To get the most from corneal tomography, every detail, value, digit, maps, and profiles should be understood and correlated to clinical findings. In other words, a tomographic-clinical matrix is the aim of this book.

This book is the practical application of the 4th edition of the mother book "Corneal Tomography in Clinical Practice." Therefore, the readers are advised to read that book in conjunction with this book for better understanding.

This edition is much different from the previous two editions in several points. This edition standardizes the method of capturing the cornea and excluding the sources of false findings. This edition presents two new algorithms, the practical subjective scoring system (PS3) for laser-based refractive surgery and the practical subjective IOL selection (PSIS) for lens-based refractive surgery. It represents the new categorization of the ectatic corneal diseases, correlates the tomographic findings with their clinical applications, and highlights the importance of corneal wavefront in decision making. This edition presents the parameters, rules, and work up of laser-based and lens-based refractive surgery as well as cataract surgery. It discusses four clinical cases in a systematic method.

Mazen M Sinjab

Preface to the First Edition

Taking the right decision in laser refractive surgery depends to a great extent on good reading of corneal topography and its clinical interpretation. This is very important for having the aimed results and avoiding postoperative complications.

Data in this book were obtained and gathered from the user manual of the Pentacam, international conferences, refractive journals, personal contacts with many refractive professors and, of course, self-experience.

The strategy in compiling this little book is making a quick refreshment of what has been explained in the previous book "Corneal Topography in Clinical Practice" published by M/s Jaypee Brothers Medical Publishers (P) Ltd, New Delhi, India and then follows a systematic approach of topographical pictures in chosen cases. This strategy allows the readers to qualify and quantify any case in the future in a way that no data may be lost.

There are sure to be some errors. As the ophthalmology editor, I take the full responsibility for these and look forward to being further educated.

Mazen M Sinjab

Contents

Abbreviations

AB	Asymmetric Bowtie
AC	Anterior Chamber
ACA	Anterior Chamber Angle
ACD	Anterior Chamber Depth
AK	Astigmatic Keratotomy
ATR	Against-the-rule
BAD	Belin-Ambrosio Display
BFS	Best Fit Sphere
BFTE	Best Fit Toric Ellipsoid
CAD	Central Ablation Depth
CCT	Central Corneal Thickness
CDVA	Corrected Distance Visual Acuity
CI	Confidence Interval
CLE	Clear Lens Extraction
CLVC	Customized Laser Vision Correction
CTSP	Corneal Thickness Spatial Profile
CXL	Corneal Crosslinking
DED	Dry Eye Disease
DOF	Depth of Focus
ECDs	Ectatic Corneal Diseases
EDOF	Extended Depth of Focus
EKR	Equivalent K-reading
ELP	EFfective Lens Position
EMEs	Entities Misdiagnosed as Ectasia
Epi-LASIK	Epipolis Laser in situ Keratomileusis
FemtoLASIK	Femtosecond Laser in situ Keratomileusis
FFKC	Forme Fruste Keratoconus

FT	Flap Thickness
HOAs	Higher-order Aberrations
HSTS	Horizontal Sulcus-to-sulcus
HWTW	Horizontal White-to-white
ICRs	Intracorneal Rings
IOL	Intraocular Lens
KC	Keratoconus
KCS	Keratoconus Suspect
KG	Keratoglobus
Km	Mean K-reading
Kmax	Maximum K-reading
LASEK	Laser Subepithelial Keratomileusis
LASIK	Laser in situ Keratomileusis
LRIs	Limbal Relaxing Incisions
LVC	Laser Vision Correction
MA	Manifest Astigmatism
OSD	Ocular Surface Disease
OZ	Optical Zone
PIOL	Phakic Intraocular Lens
PLK	Pellucid-like Keratoconus
PMD	Pellucid Marginal Degeneration
PRK	Photorefractive Keratectomy
PS3	The Practical Subjective Scoring System
PSIS	The Practical Subjective IOL Selection
PTA	Percent Tissue Altered
PTI	Percentage Thickness Increase
Qs	Quality Specifications
RLE	Refractive Lens Exchange
RMS	Root Mean Square
SA	Spherical Aberration
SB	Symmetric Bowtie

SBK	Sub-Bowman Keratomileusis
SE	Spherical Equivalent
SIA	Surgically-induced Astigmatism
Sim-Ks	Simulated Keratometric Readings
SMILE	Small Incision Lenticule Extraction
SRAX	Skewed Radial Axis Index
TA	Tomographic Astigmatism
TCRP	Total Corneal Refractive Power
TCT	Thinnest Corneal Thickness
TE-PRK	Transepithelial Photorefractive Keratectomy
TR	Total Refraction
TZ	Treated Zone
UDVA	Uncorrected Distance Visual Acuity
WTR	With-the-rule

Introduction

TEN PEARLS BEFORE READING CORNEAL TOMOGRAPHY

1. Decision making in refractive surgery is based not only on corneal tomography but on other investigations as well.
2. Reading corneal tomography should follow a systematic method and should depend on reading and interpreting as many maps and profiles as possible.
3. Tomographical findings should alert the surgeon to re-examine the patient more carefully as some clinical findings may be overlooked.
4. Abnormal or unusual tomographic findings should alert the technician and the surgeon to look for the sources of false findings and to recapture the patient.
5. The cut-off values presented in this book are evidence-based unless there is a notification where personal communications are the source of information.
6. The specificity and sensitivity of the cut-off values are variable because of the false positives and false negatives.
7. Some of the cut-off values differ according to populations. For example, some populations may have normal thin corneas, while other populations may have bilateral symmetric inferior, superior asymmetry. Therefore, the cut-off values should be personalized according to the population.
8. Corneal tomography findings should be interpreted in correlation with the clinical findings.

9. Ectatic corneal disorders (ECDs) have tomographic terminology that should be well understood and followed to differentiate the ECDs from other corneal irregularities, especially those occurring after laser-based refractive surgery.

10. To understand this book and practice it efficiently, readers are advised to read the latest versions of the author's two books: *Corneal Tomography in Clinical Practice* and *Five Steps To Start Your Refractive Surgery*.

Standardize the Capture: Screening Guidelines

■ THE 4-COMPOSITE REFRACTIVE MAP

Study the 4-composite refractive map that consists of the anterior curvature sagittal map, the anterior and posterior elevation maps, and the thickness map **(Fig. 1.1)**. Adjust the settings of the device to get standard captures.

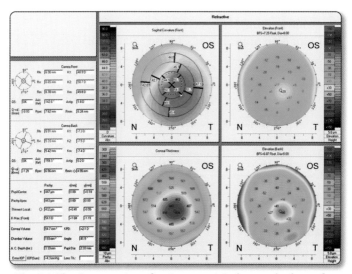

Fig. 1.1: The 4-composite refractive map. It is the standard map for refractive and cataract study.

■ GENERAL SETTINGS (FIG. 1.2)

- K-value presentation. Choose "mm" for the unit and "R hor./R vert." for the type of display.
- Axis of astigmatism. Choose "Flat Meridian". The flat meridian will be displayed in blue and the steep meridian in red.
- The box of "Show sign of Astigmatism" should be left blank.
- Store 9 mm Zone setting.
- Shape Factor Presentation. Choose "Asphericity (Q)."
- Eccentricity Calculation Zone. Choose "Peripheral mm-Rings," "20 Sag. Angle Ring," and "6 mm-ring (Dia)."
- Elevation Reference Shape. Choose "sphere," "float," "optimize shift" and "Manual 8 mm."
- Anterior Chamber Depth Range. Choose "Internal (Endothelium)."
- Color Map Appearance. Choose "Black Dots."

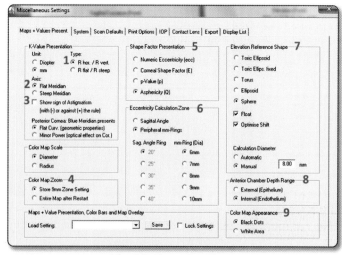

Fig. 1.2: General settings.

■ MAIN COLOR BAR SETTINGS (FIG. 1.3)

- *Curvature Color Bar:* Tick the options, as shown in the figure. Although 'Belin Intuitive' is recommended as a color pattern, the reader can use any color pattern.
- *Pachy Color Bar:* Tick the options, as shown in the figure. Although Ambrosio2 is recommended as a color pattern, the reader can use any color pattern.
- *Elevation Color Bar:* Tick the options, as shown in the figure. Although Belin Intuitive is recommended as a color pattern, the reader can use any color pattern.

■ MAPS OVERLAY

The map overlay consists of the components that should appear on the maps. Right-click on each of the four maps to open the corresponding box of options.

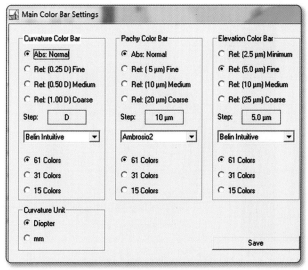

Fig. 1.3: Main color bar settings.

- *Sagittal Curvature (Front):* Tick the options, as shown in **Figure 1.4**. Note that "Min. Radius Pos. Front" is the maximum K reading (Kmax) on the anterior corneal surface (**Fig. 1.5** red arrow).

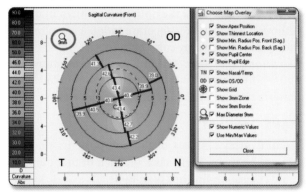

Fig. 1.4: Overlay of the anterior sagittal curvature map.

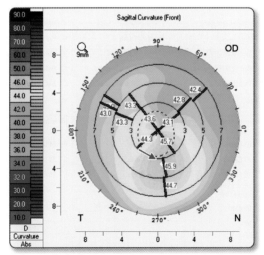

Fig. 1.5: Symbol of Kmax on the anterior sagittal curvature.

- *Elevation Maps:* Tick the options, as shown in **Figure 1.6**.
- *Thickness Map Overlay:* Tick the options, as shown in **Figure 1.7**.

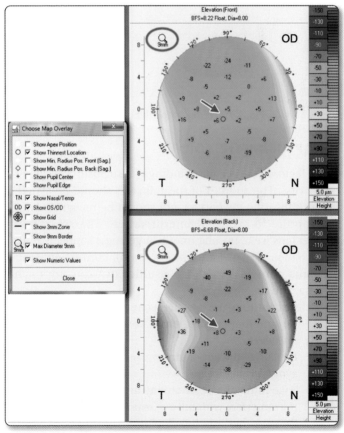

Fig. 1.6: Overlay of the elevation maps.

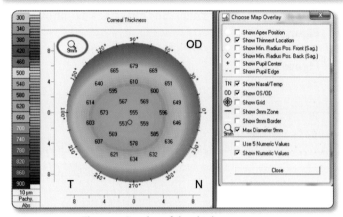

Fig. 1.7: Overlay of the thickness map.

■ CAPTURING THE CORNEA

Some factors produce false findings (false positives and false negatives). The sources of these factors should be avoided before capturing the cornea and should be recognized after the capture to avoid misinterpretation. The sources are contact lens wear, misalignment, large angle kappa, tear film disturbance (dry eye and excess tears), corneal opacities, previous corneal surgeries, insufficient exposure to the camera, and pregnancy.

- Before capturing the eye, the technician should:
  1. Be sure that contact lenses were stopped for at least one week.
  2. Explain to the patient the proper method of fixation to avoid misalignment.
  3. Take into consideration any anatomical features that may interfere with full eye exposure to the camera.
  4. Be sure that any headcover, including head scarfs, should be aside from the camera pathway.

5. Alert the physician if the patient is pregnant, has dry eye symptoms, had a history of eye infection (source of corneal scars or opacities), or has a history of previous corneal surgery.

- While taking the capture, the technician:
  1. Should align the device properly.
  2. Should monitor the eye continuously.
  3. Must *not* use anesthesia drops. If the technician finds the patient blinking frequently, dry eye is suspected. Anesthesia drops are forbidden because they alter the integrity of the epithelium, tear film, and corneal surface.
  4. Should *not* using lubricant drops immediately before the capture. Dry eye disease should sufficiently be treated before the exam.

■ VALIDATING THE QUALITY OF THE CAPTURE

After taking the capture, there are two steps for validating the quality of the captures. The first step is performed by the technician before printing the exam, and the second step is performed by the physician when they receive the printed exam.

Technician Step

Before printing the capture and sending it to the physician, the technician should validate the capture by the following steps:

1. *Quality specification (Qs):* It should be white "OK."
2. No extrapolated area in the 9-mm display. If there is extrapolation **(Fig. 1.8)**, the capture should be repeated.
3. *Km:* Three captures should be taken in the session. The Km (mean K reading on the anterior corneal surface) is compared. If >0.3 D difference is found between the

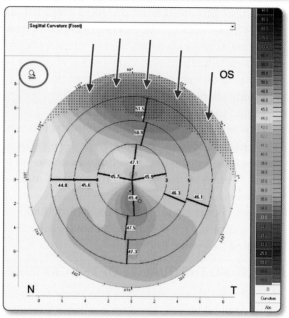

Fig. 1.8: Extrapolation due to missed data. The arrows indicate a black-dotted zone of extrapolated data in the 9-mm display.

captures, they should be repeated. If the difference is insignificant, the capture with the median number is reliable. *Example 1:* Three captures with Km 45.3 D, 45.8 D, and 45 D; the captures should be repeated. *Example 2:* Three captures with Km 43.4 D, 43.7 D, and 43.5 D; the captures are accepted, and the median one (43.5 D) is the reliable capture for this visit. That is important, especially in observing the progression of ectatic corneal diseases (ECDs) and comparing pre- with postoperative results. Please note that the variation in Km is high in ectatic eyes, hence the need to be patient while taking the captures.

4. *Kmax:* Check the symbol of the maximum K-reading (Kmax) on the anterior sagittal map. If it is very peripheral (**Fig. 1.9** red arrow), recapture the cornea; if it is repeatedly peripheral, check lid position on Scheimpflug images; if there is no lid interference, tell the physician to check tear film and look for blepharitis, inferior punctate epithelial erosions, or corneal scars.

5. *Misalignment:* To rule out misalignment and differentiate it from large angle kappa, compare X and Y coordinates of pupil center between the two eyes. Usually, the sign of X is –ve in the right eye and +ve in the left eye, and vice versa in case of negative angle Kappa (e.g., high axial myopia). On the other hand, the sign of Y should be similar in both eyes, i.e., both –ve or both +ve. To check misalignment,

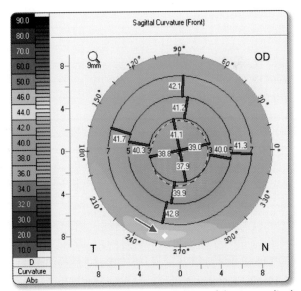

Fig. 1.9: Kmax symbol at the very periphery of the 9-mm display.

calculate $X + X$, and $Y - Y$. If $X + X$ and/or $Y - Y$ >0.2 mm (> 200 μm), there is misalignment (**Fig. 1.10** red arrows) and the capture should be repeated. On the other hand, angle kappa is symmetric in both eyes regardless of its value. **Figure 1.11** is an example of a large angle kappa. In the case of large angle kappa, an abnormal skewed radial axis index (SRAX) can be considered insignificant and can be neglected.

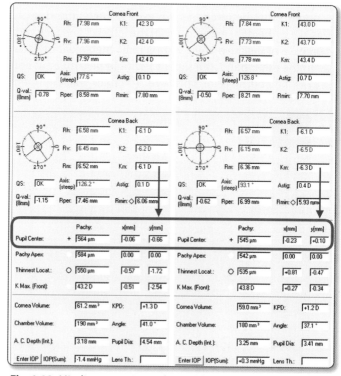

Fig. 1.10: Misalignment. A significant difference in the pupil-center y-coordinate between two eyes.

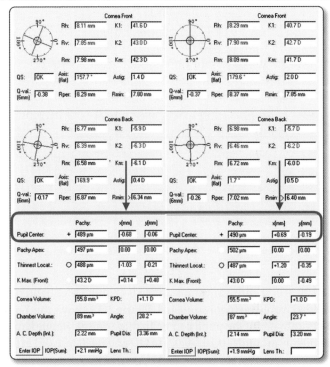

Fig. 1.11: Large angle kappa. Inter-eye symmetric coordinates of the pupil center.

It is essential to know that the Pentacam does not measure angle kappa directly. There are two methods to estimate the angle by the Pentacam, chord μ in the Holladay report, and considering half the values of X and Y coordinates of pupil center if Holladay report is not available. **Figure 1.12** is the Holladay report measuring chord μ (red ellipse). It is the chord distance from vertex normal (assumed to be the visual axis) and the pupil center. On the Pentacam, the normal value

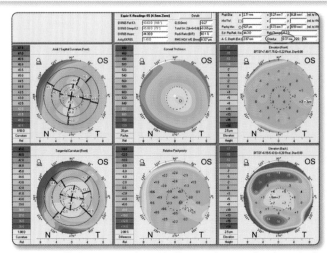

Fig. 1.12: Holladay report. The red ellipse indicates Chord μ, which is an approximation of angle kappa.

is 0.20 ± 0.11 mm, so values above 0.42 mm (highlighted in yellow) would be highly unusual. **Figure 1.13** shows the X and Y coordinates of the pupil center. In this example, angle kappa is roughly around (−0.10, +0.02) in OD and (−0.02, −0.05) in OS.

Physician Step

The physician should check the followings before accepting the capture:

1. Check Qs. Qs should be white "OK."
2. Check if any extrapolated area in the 9-mm display, as mentioned above.
3. Check misalignment, as described above.
4. Check astigmatic disparity. Compare tomographic astigmatism (TA) with the subjective manifest astigmatism (MA). The best way to measure TA is the total corneal refractive power (TCRP) at the 3-mm ring centered

	Pachy:	x[mm]	y[mm]		Pachy:	x[mm]	y[mm]
Pupil Center:	+ 559 µm	-0.20	+0.04	Pupil Center:	+ 563 µm	-0.04	-0.11
Pachy Apex:	· 560 µm	0.00	0.00	Pachy Apex:	564 µm	0.00	0.00
Thinnest Locat.:	O 548 µm	-0.96	-0.82	Thinnest Locat.:	O 556 µm	+0.33	-0.99
K Max. (Front):	44.9 D	+0.21	+1.17	K Max. (Front):	45.2 D	-0.07	-0.99
	OD				OS		

Fig. 1.13: Pupil center coordinates relative to corneal apex.

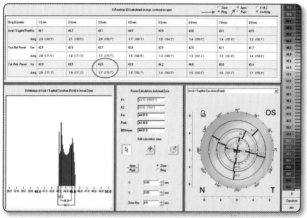

Fig. 1.14: The total corneal refractive power (TCRP) in the power display. The red arrows indicate the standard settings: ring/apex. The red ellipse indicates the true total corneal astigmatism measured by the TCRP at 3-mm ring/apex.

with the apex **(Fig. 1.14)**. If that is not available, it can be calculated roughly by deducting the magnitude of posterior astigmatism from the anterior one **(Fig. 1.15)** and using the *flat* anterior axis. Please note that the sign of astigmatism should not be displayed to avoid confusion. In **Figure 1.15**, the anterior astigmatism is 4.7 D, and the posterior astigmatism is 0.9 D, therefore TA = 4.7 – 0.9 = 3.8 D × 3.3° (the *flat* axis of anterior astigmatism). This TA should be compared with the MA using the absolute value at the flat axis.

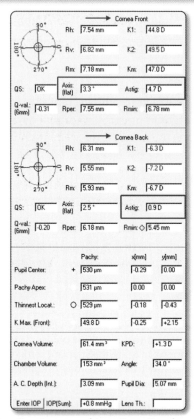

Fig. 1.15: Estimating tomographic astigmatism by subtracting the absolute values of the posterior from the anterior astigmatism and using the flat axis of the anterior astigmatism.

A difference of ≥1 D in magnitude or ≥10° in axis is considered abnormal; thus, the capture should be repeated. If the disparity continues to appear in the following captures, exclude early cataract, corneal opacities, and other sources of false findings.

Read in a Systematic Method: The Systematic Interpretation of Corneal Tomography

This chapter discusses the systematic interpretation of the 4-composite refractive map and the complimentary maps and profiles.

INTERPRETATION OF THE 4-COMPOSITE REFRACTIVE MAP (FIG. 2.1)

There are six points to look at in this map. The author classifies the six points into low risk (normal), moderate risk (suspicious), and high risk in terms of corneal refractive surgery.

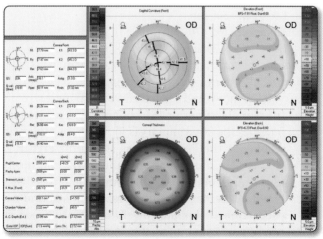

Fig. 2.1: The 4-composite refractive map.

1. *Km (mean K) of the anterior corneal surface (**Fig. 2.2** red ellipse):* The cut-off value of Km is 48 in the Pentacam and 47.2 D in placido-based devices.
   - *Low risk:* <48 D.
   - *Moderate risk:* 48–50 D.
   - *High risk:* >50 D.

2. *The thinnest corneal thickness (**Fig. 2.2** blue ellipse):* In general, many factors affect corneal thickness, such as age, gender, environmental and genetic factors, race, ocular pressure, corneal pathologies, and diabetes, in addition to diurnal variation.

   Based on an international study, the mean thinnest-point pachymetry was 536 µm overall, and values less than 469 or 435 µm (–2 or –3 SD, respectively) would be expected in less than 2.5% or 0.15% of normal corneas, respectively. Although some populations may have thinner corneas, the author considers the –2 SD as a cut-off value for safety measures.
   - *Low risk:* >500 µm.
   - *Moderate risk:* 470–500 µm.
   - *High risk:* <470 µm.

3. *Anterior sagittal map:* The anterior sagittal map is studied in terms of inferior, superior asymmetry, skewed radial axis (SRAX) index, and sagittal curvature patterns.
   (a) Inferior (I), superior (S) asymmetry. The standard index for the IS asymmetry is shown in the topometric display in the Pentacam, as shown in **Figure 2.3** (red arrow). According to Rabinowitz, the normal IS is <1.5 D; otherwise, it is abnormal. If this display is not available, the author recommends and easy estimation. Calculate the difference between the two opposing points on the steep vertical axis in the 4-mm zone (the two red ellipses). Consider I-S if I > S,

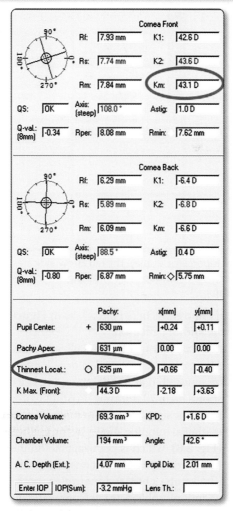

Fig. 2.2: The data of the 4-composite refractive map. The red ellipse indicates the mean K-reading on the anterior corneal surface (Km). The blue ellipse indicates the thickness at the thinnest location.

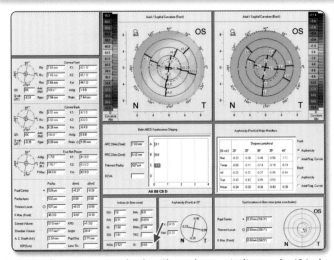

Fig. 2.3: The topometric display. The red arrow indicates the IS index, representing the inferior, superior asymmetry on the anterior sagittal curvature map.

as in **Figure 2.4**, or S-I if S > I, as in **Figure 2.5**. Based on the author's method:

- *Low risk:* I–S <1.5 D or S–I <2.5 D.
- *Moderate risk:* I–S ≥ 1.5 D or S–I ≥ 2.5 D. This can be ignored, if epithelial mapping is available and shows no focal thinning. In other words, the asymmetry is significant only if associated with focal epithelial thinning shown by the epithelial mapping **(Fig. 2.6)**, which is not available on the Pentacam. Moreover, some populations have inferior, superior asymmetry, but symmetric in both eyes as in enantiomorphism. In such populations, the inferior, superior asymmetry is considered insignificant as long as this asymmetry is bilateral and identical.
- No high risk.

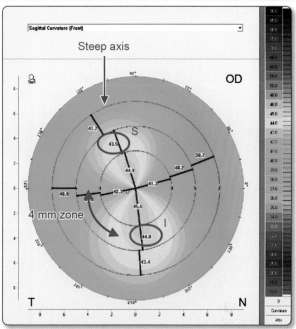

Fig. 2.4: The anterior sagittal curvature map. The red ellipses indicate the two opposing points on the steep axis in the 4-mm zone (the second circle of numbers). The difference in value represents the inferior, superior asymmetry. In this image, the inferior value is larger than the superior one.

Please note that the author's method is more accurate in with-the-rule (WTR) astigmatism rather than oblique and against-the-rule (ATR) astigmatism because the steep axis in the last two is not vertical.

(b) *Skewed radial axis index (SRAX) in the steep inner segments (**Fig. 2.7** red arrows):*
- *Low risk:* SRAX < 22°.
- *Moderate risk:* No moderate risk.

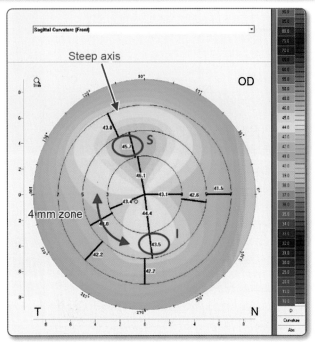

Fig. 2.5: The anterior sagittal curvature map. The red ellipses indicate the two opposing points on the steep axis in the 4-mm zone (the second circle of numbers). The difference in value represents the inferior and superior asymmetry. In this image, the superior value is larger than the inferior one.

- *High risk:* SRAX ≥ 22° and tomographic astigmatism (TA) ≥1 D. If the TA is <1 D, SRAX is considered insignificant, as in **Figure 2.8**. In the case of large angle kappa, a bilateral symmetric SRAX is considered insignificant.
(c) *Pattern:* Butterfly, crab claw, vertical D, and clown face are at high risk **(Fig. 2.9)**.

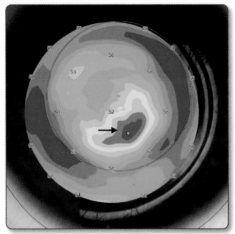

Fig. 2.6: Epithelial thickness map. This map is not available in the Pentacam. The black arrow indicates the focal thinning pattern.

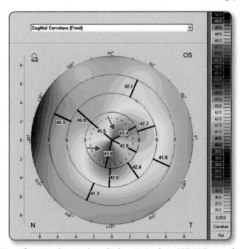

Fig. 2.7: Significant skewed radial axis index (SRAX) on the anterior sagittal curvature map. The red arrows indicate the inner segments representing the skewing.

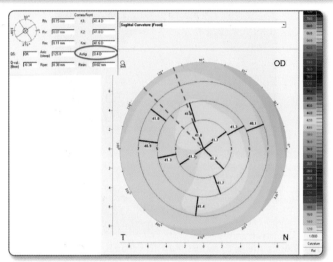

Fig. 2.8: Insignificant skewed radial axis index (SRAX) because the topographic astigmatism is <1 D.

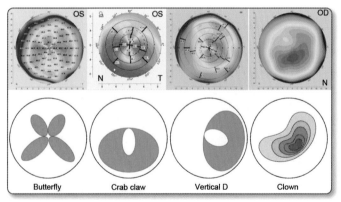

Fig. 2.9: Patterns of high-risk on the anterior sagittal curvature map.

4. *Elevation Maps:* There are two different methods in evaluating the elevation maps, the Best Fit Sphere (BFS) and the Best Fit Toric Ellipsoid (BFTE), both in float optimize shift mode with manual 8 mm diameter. The BFS is recommended by Michael Belin and Renato Ambrosio, while the BFTE is recommended by Jack Holladay.

In the BFS method, look at the values corresponding to the thinnest location.

- *Low risk (**Fig. 2.10**):*
  - <8 µm on anterior, <18 µm on posterior in emmetropia and myopia.
  - <7 µm on anterior, <28 µm on posterior in hyperopia and mixed astigmatism.
- No moderate risk.
- *High risk (**Fig. 2.11**):*
  - ≥8 µm on anterior, ≥18 µm on posterior in emmetropia and myopia.
  - ≥7 µm on anterior, ≥28 µm on posterior in hyperopia and mixed astigmatism.

In the BFTE method, look at the values in the central 5-mm zone.

- *Low risk (**Fig. 2.12**):* ≤12 µm on anterior, ≤15 µm on posterior regardless of the refraction.
- No moderate risk.
- *High risk (**Fig. 2.13**):* >12 µm on anterior, >15 µm on posterior regardless of the refraction.

5. *Thickness Maps:* The author depends on the pattern rather than the numeric evaluation of the thickness map.
- *Low risk:* Concentric shape **(Fig. 2.14)**.
- *Moderate risk:* Dome and droplet shapes **(Fig. 2.15)**.
- *High risk:* Bell and Globus shapes **(Fig. 2.16)**.

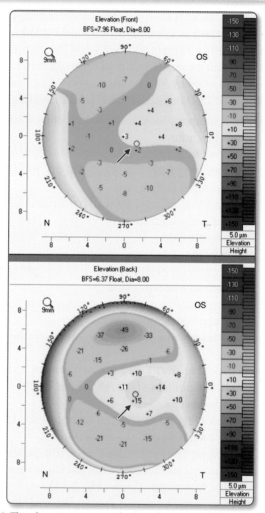

Fig. 2.10: The elevation maps in the best fit sphere, float, optimize shift, 8-mm diameter mode. The red arrows point at the values corresponding to the thinnest location. This is an example of low-risk values.

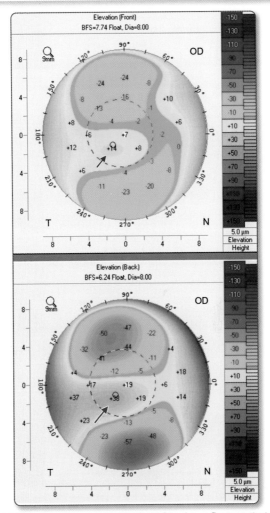

Fig. 2.11: The elevation maps in the best fit sphere, float, optimize shift, 8-mm diameter mode. The red arrows point at the values corresponding to the thinnest location. This is an example of high-risk values.

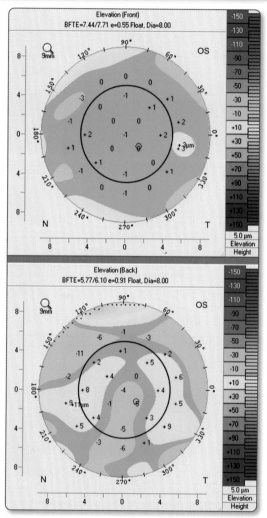

Fig. 2.12: The elevation maps in the best fit toric ellipsoid, float, optimize shift, 8-mm diameter mode. The black circles represent the central 5-mm zone. This is an example of low-risk values.

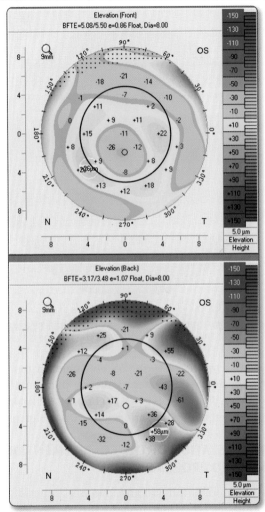

Fig. 2.13: The elevation maps in the best fit toric ellipsoid, float, optimize shift, 8-mm diameter mode. The black circles represent the central 5-mm zone. This is an example of high-risk values.

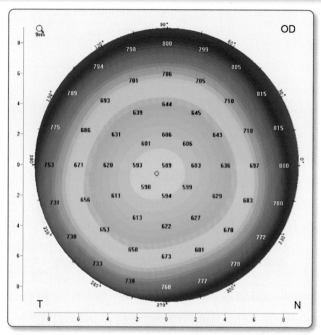

Fig. 2.14: The concentric pattern of the thickness map.

6. *Inter-eye asymmetry Maps:* Follow **Table 2.1** to compare between both eyes in terms of five parameters. Each parameter, if positive, is given a score of 1. If the total score is 4, it is a moderate risk, and if it is 5, it is a high risk.

INTERPRETATION OF THE COMPLEMENTARY MAPS AND PROFILES

In daily practice, physicians usually depend on the 4-composite refractive map because they do not have access to other maps. However, if other maps are available, the study would be more accurate and more reliable.

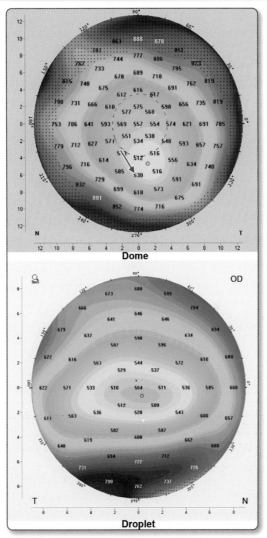

Fig. 2.15: The dome and droplet shapes of the thickness map.

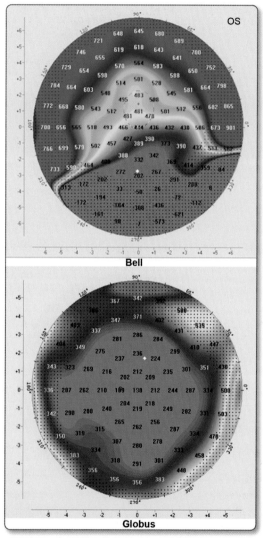

Fig. 2.16: The bell and globus shapes of the thickness map.

Table 2.1: Intereye corneal asymmetry score.[a]

Scoring Criteria	Positive (+1 point) if Intereye Difference
Mean anterior keratometry (Km anterior)	≥0.3 D
Mean posterior keratometry (Km posterior)	≥0.1 D
Thinnest pachymetry	≥12 μm
Front elevation at thinnest location	≥2 μm
Back elevation at thinnest location	≥5 μm

[a]Score of 3 is observed in up to 6–11% of healthy patients, whereas a score of 4 is found in less than 4% of patients without keratoconus. A score of 5 should be considered highly abnormal (1% or less of non-keratoconic patients).

Pachymetry Profiles: Corneal Thickness Spatial Profile (CTSP) and Percentage Thickness Increase (PTI)

The normal pattern of both CTSP and PTI is a curved line plotted in red, following (but not necessarily within) the course of the normative black-dotted curves, with an average less than 1.20 (**Fig. 2.17** blue arrow). In other words, the shape of the curve should show gradual increment. The reference in this regard is the 6-mm zone (**Fig. 2.17** red circles). If the curve deviates before this zone, it is considered abnormal.

Abnormal patterns are:
- *Quick slope (Fig. 2.18):* The red curve declines before the 6-mm zone. It is encountered in ECDs and corneas with high potential to develop ectasia, if operated (See Chapter 3).
- *S-shape:* After descending, the red curve ascends. The ascending might be before the 6-mm zone (**Fig. 2.19**), or after it (**Fig. 2.20**). This pattern is usually seen in ECDs and corneas with high potential.

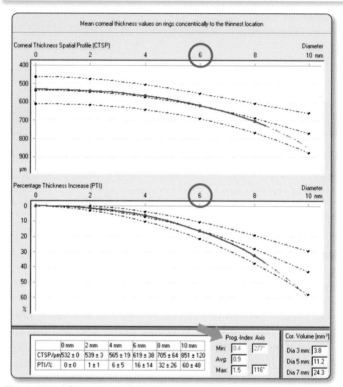

Fig. 2.17: Pachymetry profiles. The red circles indicate the 6-mm zone relative to the thinnest location. The 6-mm zone is a reference to describe the shape of the curves. The blue arrow indicates the average of thickness progression.

- *Flat slope (Fig. 2.21):* It is usually seen in diseased thickened corneas, such as corneal edema, Fuchs' endothelial dystrophy, and cornea guttata. However, the absence of this sign does not exclude the diagnosis.
- *Inverted slope (Fig. 2.22):* It is a hallmark of PMD. However, not every PMD has this pattern.

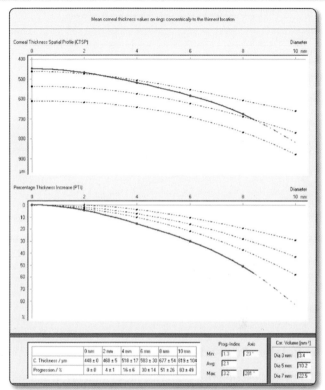

Fig. 2.18: Quick slop pattern of the pachymetry profiles.

Regarding the average, as mentioned above, it normally is <1.2. However, if it is ≥1.2 and all other parameters are within the low-risk category, it can be ignored because it is common to see a high average associated with high corneal astigmatism (>2 D), especially mixed astigmatism. Therefore, look for all risk factors, if all are at low risk except the average and there is high corneal astigmatism, consider the high average a low-risk factor rather than a moderate one.

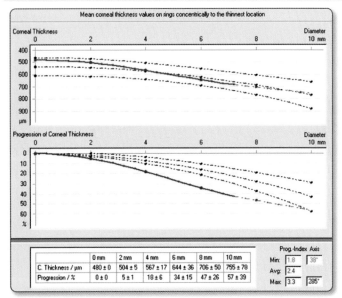

Fig. 2.19: S-shape before the 6-mm zone in the pachymetry profiles.

The Relative Pachymetry Map

The first to describe this map was Jack Holladay. It is used in the Holladay report. According to Holladay, the map is normal if all the values are >–5% (e.g. –2%) all over the 9-mm display. The map is suspicious if any value is between –5% and –8%, and abnormal if any value is <–8% (e.g. –12%).

This map is essential in detecting a previous corneal surgery, and in differentiating ECDs from entities mimicking ECDs.

Based on the author's observation, many cases of normal corneas fall in between –5% and –8%. Therefore, this map is normal (low risk) when all values are > –8% (e.g., –6%),

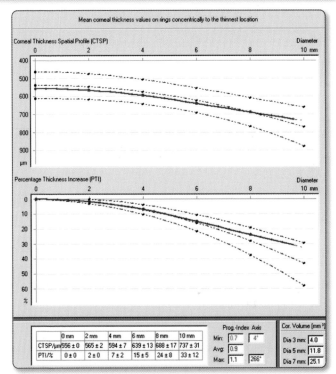

Fig. 2.20: S-shape after the 6-mm zone in the pachymetry profiles.

as in **Figure 2.23**, and this map is suspicious (moderate risk) when any value is ≤8% (e.g., -9%), as in **Figure 2.24**.

Belin Ambrosio Display (BAD)

The BAD is an elevation-based classification system developed by Michael Belin and Renato Ambrosio for the early detection of ECDs. The BAD depends on the principle of "Enhanced Best Fit Sphere."

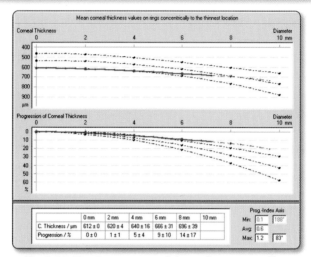

Fig. 2.21: Flat slope pattern of the pachymetry profiles.

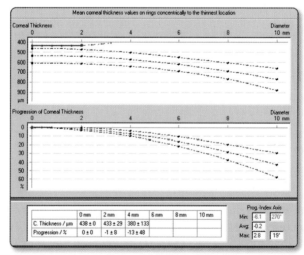

Fig. 2.22: The inverted slope pattern of the pachymetry profiles.

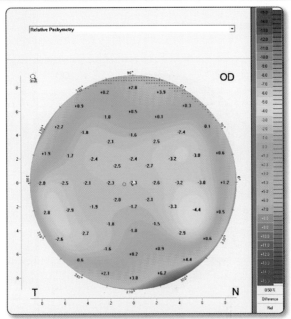

Fig. 2.23: The relative pachymetry map.
This is an example of a normal map.

The BAD consists of OD and OS columns. Each column consists of three maps. The map on the bottom is the display of interest. If the display (the map on the bottom) is green **(Fig. 2.25)**, the elevation maps are normal; if the display has a yellow flag **(Fig. 2.26)**, the elevation maps are suspicious; and if the display has a red flag **(Fig. 2.27** bottom right), the maps are abnormal.

The BAD gives an idea about the elevation maps and enhance the screening, but should not be considered a definite diagnostic display because of false negatives and false positives, and because it is elevation-based and does not

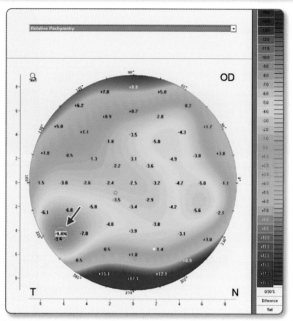

Fig. 2.24: The relative pachymetry map. This is an example of an abnormal map. The red arrow indicates the area of abnormal value.

consider the curvature maps and the thickness map. There are four sources of false positives in BAD: large angle kappa, misalignment, corneal scars, and corneal pathologies.

■ EXCLUDING FACTORS OF FALSE FINDINGS

As mentioned in Chapter 1, several factors have an impact on the reliability of corneal tomography. They are responsible for false positives (false *abnormal* findings) and false negatives (false *normal* findings). False positives may cause over-estimating and excluding suitable candidates for refractive surgery, while false negatives may cause under-estimating

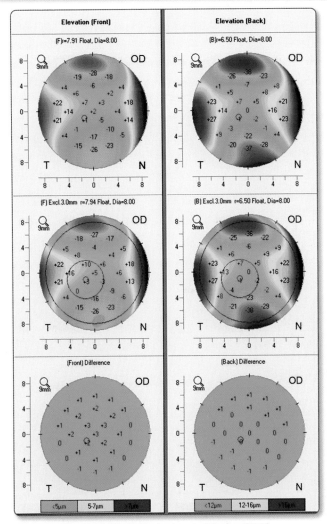

Fig. 2.25: The Belin Ambrosio Display (BAD).
An example of normal display.

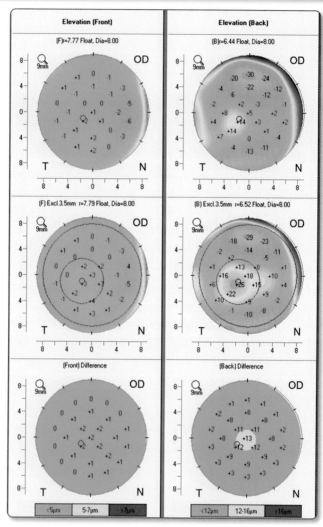

Fig. 2.26: The Belin Ambrosio Display (BAD).
An example of suspicious display.

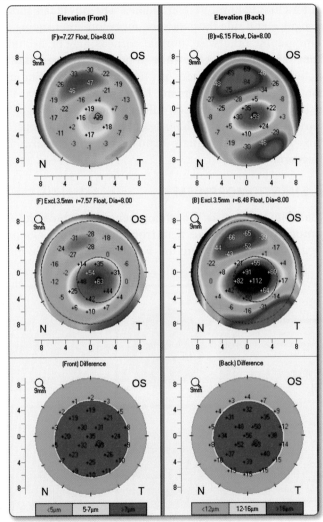

Fig. 2.27: The Belin Ambrosio Display (BAD).
An example of abnormal display.

and including improper candidates. The physician should recognize and rule these factors out before interpreting the tomography; otherwise, normal corneas may be excluded from refractive surgery, while abnormal corneas may be included. In general, there are 10 sources of false findings: contact lenses, misalignment, large angle kappa, tear film disturbance, ocular surface inflammation and pathologies, corneal opacities and pathologies, previous corneal surgeries, early cataract, inadequate exposure to the camera, and pregnancy.

■ ENANTIOMORPHISM

Enantiomorphism is the phenomenon in which the OD tomography looks like a mirror image of the OS one. **Figures 2.28 and 2.29** are the 4-composite refractive maps

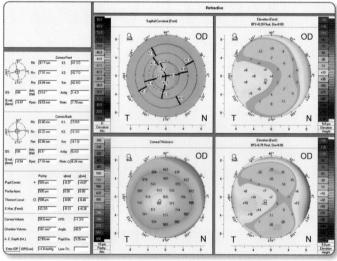

Fig. 2.28: Enantiomorphism. The right eye.

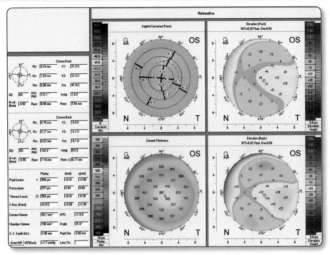

Fig. 2.29: Enantiomorphism. The left eye.

of a refractive surgery candidate. These figures are a typical example of this phenomenon. Enantiomorphism is useful to accept the SRAX when it is abnormal and to accept I-S asymmetry in some populations, if not associated with epithelial thinning.

THE PRACTICAL SUBJECTIVE SCORING SYSTEM (PS3) ALGORITHM

Table 2.2 summarizes the Practical Subjective Scoring System (PS3), which classifies the tomographic risk factors into low (normal), moderate (suspicious), and high-risk factors regarding laser-based refractive surgery. The intuitive low-risk factors will not be displayed in **Table 2.2**. The PS3 was established by the author based on the cut-off values and patterns mentioned above. **Table 2.3** represents the author's method in applying the PS3 on candidate selection based on

Table 2.2: The practical subjective scoring system.

Parameters	Moderate Risk	High risk
Anterior Km (D)	48–50	>50
Thinnest Location (μm)	470–500[a]	<470[a]
Anterior Sagittal Map	• I–S ≥ 1.5 D if I > S[b] • S–I ≥ 2.5 D if S > I[b]	• SRAX ≥ 22° [c] • Butterfly, crab claw, vertical D, and clown face
Elevation Maps based on BFS	–	• ≥ +8 μm anterior or ≥ +18 μm posterior in emmetropia and myopia • ≥ +7 μm anterior or ≥ +28 μm posterior in hyperopia and mixed astigmatism
Elevation Maps based on BFTE	–	>+12 μm anterior or >+15 μm posterior, regardless of refraction
Corneal Thickness Map	Dome and Droplet	Bell and Globus
Thickness Profiles	• Normal slope but average ≥1.20[d] • S shape after 6 mm	• Quick slope • S shape before 6 mm • Inverted slope
Relative Thickness Map	<–8% (e.g. –12%)	-
Inter-Eye Asymmetry	Score 4	Score 5

(Km: mean K-reading; TCT: thinnest corneal thickness; BFS: Best fit sphere; BFTE: Best fit toric ellipsoid; SRAX: skewed radial axis index; SE: spherical equivalent)
[a]Can be modified according to population
[b]Can be ignored if not associated with focal epithelial thinning
[c]Can be ignored if tomographic astigmatism is <1 D and in the case of enantiomorphism
[d]Can be ignored if all other tomographic features are normal and corneal astigmatism is >2 D.

corneal tomography. It is essential to exclude sources of false findings before applying the PS3 to avoid overestimation or underestimation. In other words, all the steps of avoiding and recognizing the false findings should be mastered to

Table 2.3: Application of the practical subjective scoring system on laser-based refractive surgery.

	Low Risk	*One Moderate*	*Two Moderate or One High*
Suface Ablation	✓	✓	X
SMILE[a]	✓	✓	X
LASIK[b]	✓	X	X

[a]Small Incision Lenticule Extraction
[b]Laser In Situ Keratomileusis

be able to apply the PS3 and avoid exclusion of suitable candidates (overestimation) or include improper candidates (underestimation). As shown in **Table 2.3**:

- *No moderate- or high-risk factors in both eyes:* All types of laser-based refractive surgery are possible.
- *Two moderate- or one high-risk factor in one eye:* Both eyes are not suitable for laser-based refractive surgery.
- *One moderate risk factor in one eye, and the other eye is normal or has a moderate risk factor as well:* Both eyes are *not* suitable for LASIK.
- Please note that the PS3 is designed for laser-based, rather than lens-based, refractive surgery. Moreover, it is a tomography-based scoring system, which is a small part of the full clinical workup that the candidate must go through before making the right decision.

■ INTERPRETATION OF CORNEAL WAVEFRONT

The five higher-order aberrations (HOAs) that should be studied are mainly the spherical aberration (SA), vertical and horizontal coma, and vertical and horizontal trefoil. **Table 2.4** shows the main HOAs and their codes, according to Zernike analysis.

Table 2.4: The main higher-order aberrations.

Order	HOAs	Orientation	Code
3rd order	Coma	Vertical	Z(3, −1)
		Horizontal	Z(3, 1)
3rd order	Trefoil	Vertical	Z(3, −3)
		Horizontal	Z(3, 3)
4th order	Spherical aberration	360°	Z(4, 0)

(HOAs: higher-order aberrations)

In Zernike analysis, HOAs are measured by Zernike coefficient (ZC) and by RMS. The main difference between them is that ZC displays the HOA in negative and positive values, while the RMS is always positive. That is why it is important to look at both, especially when studying the SA to know whether it is negative or positive.

HOAs can be studied as a group or individually **(Figs. 2.30 and 2.31)**. In both cases, the settings should be adjusted to be maximum diameter = 6 mm (red ellipse) and total corneal wavefront rather than anterior or posterior surface wavefront (red arrows). In **Figure 2.30,** the aberrations are displayed as a list (blue arrow), while in **Figure 2.31**, the aberrations are displayed as a pyramid (blue arrow). In both figures, the ZC value for every individual HOA is below it, in the pyramid display, or beside it, in the list display. To study the RMS of a group of HOAs, tick the desired ones in the list, as shown in **Figure 2.30**, or click on the desired ones in the pyramid, as shown in **Figure 2.31**. Then look at the RMS of the selected HOAs (blue ellipse). This RMS is *not* a simple algebraic sum of the selected HOAs. As shown in the two figures, the main HOAs were selected. The normal value of the HOAs measured in RMS or ZC, individually and in total, is ≤ 0.35 µm (≤0.5 D).

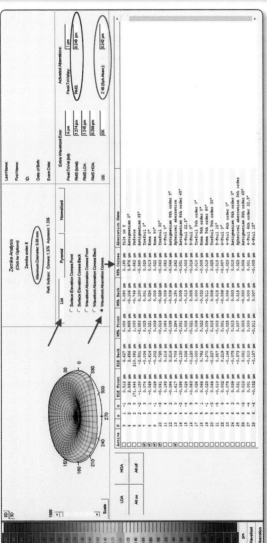

Fig. 2.30: Zernike analysis. List display. The red ellipse indicates the maximum diameter (6 mm by default). The blue arrow indicates the list option. The red arrows indicate the wavefront analysis of both corneal surfaces. The blue ellipse indicates the total RMS value of the selected aberrations. The green ellipse indicates the Zernike coefficient of the spherical aberration.

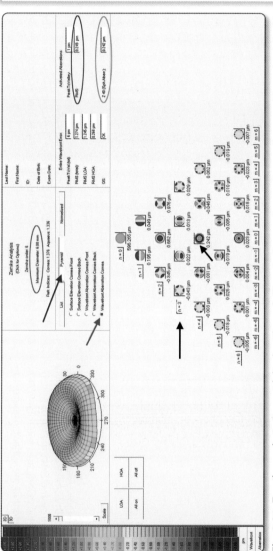

Fig. 2.31: Zernike analysis. Pyramid display. The red ellipse indicates the maximum diameter (6 mm by default). The blue arrow indicates the pyramid option. The red arrow indicates the wavefront analysis of both corneal surfaces. The black arrows indicate the five main higher-order aberrations. The blue ellipse indicates the total RMS value of the selected aberrations. The green ellipse indicates the Zernike coefficient of the spherical aberration.

The normal shape of the cornea is conoidal, which is a composition of toricity, asphericity, and asymmetry. Mathematically, asphericity can be described by eccentricity, corneal shape value (E), p-value, and Q-value. Q-value is the standard value used in this regard. The normal range of Q-value is [+0.40, –0.80], and the average range in the normal population is –0.1 to –0.3 with a mean of –0.26 **(Fig. 2.32)**. The refractive surface is called parabola or perfect prolate shape when the Q-value = –0.53, which induces no SA (zero SA) **(Fig. 2.33)**. If the Q-value is more positive, the surface is flatter, inducing +ve SA, and if the Q-value is more negative, the surface is steeper, inducing -ve SA.

Specific nomenclature is used to describe special shapes of refractive surfaces. The shapes are:

- Oblate **(Fig. 2.34)**, if Q > 0. There are +ve SA and +ve depth of focus (DOF) because the *peripheral* rays converge more than the paraxial rays to assist for near vision.

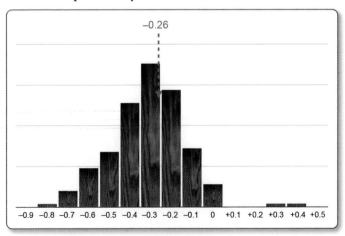

Fig. 2.32: The normal distribution of Q-value in a sample of normal population.

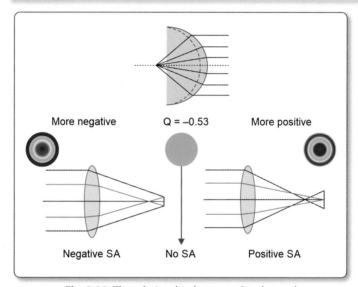

Fig. 2.33: The relationship between Q-value and spherical aberration (SA).

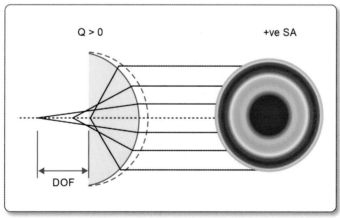

Fig. 2.34: Oblate refractive surface.

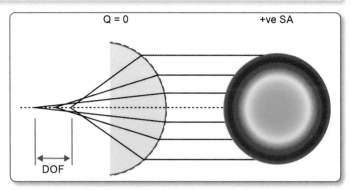

Fig. 2.35: Spherical refractive surface.

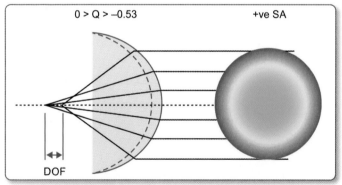

Fig. 2.36: Positive prolate refractive surface.

- Spheric **(Fig. 2.35)**, if Q = 0. There are +ve SA and +ve DOF because the *peripheral* rays converge more than the paraxial rays to assist for near vision.
- Positive prolate **(Fig. 2.36)**, if Q >–0.53 and <0. There are +ve SA and +ve DOF because the *peripheral* rays converge more than the paraxial rays to assist for near vision.
- Parabola or perfect prolate **(Fig. 2.37)**, if Q = –0.53. There is neither SA nor DOF.

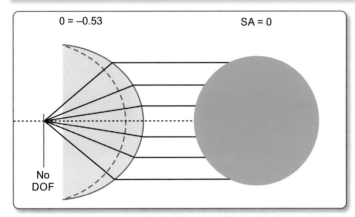

Fig. 2.37: Parabola shape (perfect prolate).

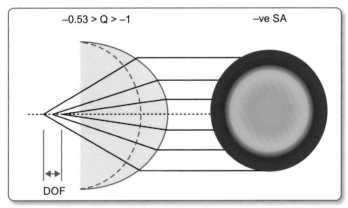

Fig. 2.38: Negative prolate refractive surface.

- Negative prolate **(Fig. 2.38)**, if Q < –0.53 and > –1. There are –ve SA and –ve DOF because the *paraxial* rays converge more than the peripheral rays to assist for near vision.
- Hyperprolate **(Fig. 2.39)**, if Q ≤ –1. There are –ve SA and –ve DOF because the *paraxial* rays converge more than the peripheral rays to assist for near vision.

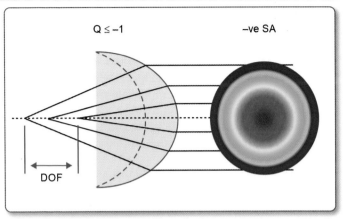

Fig. 2.39: Hyperprolate refractive surface.

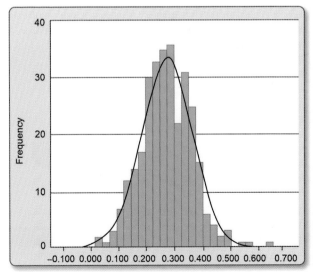

Fig. 2.40: The normal distribution of corneal spherical aberration in a sample of normal population.

Measured by ZC, the mean corneal SA in the normal population is +0.27 ± 10 μm, as shown in **Figure 2.40**. Moreover, SA can be classified into normal, non-toxic, and toxic when it is <0.35 μm, 0.35–0.6 μm, and >0.6 μm, in the –ve and +ve directions, respectively **(Fig. 2.41)**. Non-toxic means that neural adaptation can compensate for the SA without affecting the quantity of vision, while toxic means that it is out of neural adaptation capability, and the quantity of vision is affected. **Figure 2.41** shows the normal range of SA of the human cornea.

SA is beneficial in terms of the DOF that provides a depth of field for reading. The higher the SA, the larger the DOF, but that will be on account of the quality of vision because the higher the SA, the lower the contrast sensitivity, as shown in **Figure 2.42**. Moreover, the quality of vision with the –ve DOF (–ve SA) is better than with the +ve DOF (+ve SA).

Laser-based refractive surgery affects corneal asphericity. Hyperopic laser treatment converts the cornea into hyperprolate and induces –ve SA, while myopic treatment

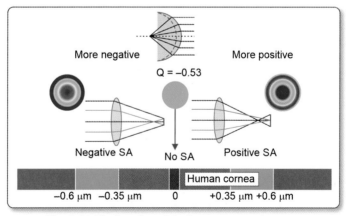

Fig. 2.41: The location of the human cornea in terms of spherical aberration (SA).

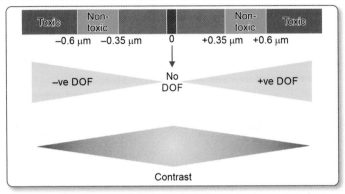

Fig. 2.42: Classification of the spherical aberration into normal, non-toxic, and toxic and the relationship with depth of focus (DOF), and contrast sensitivity.

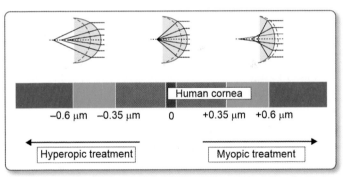

Fig. 2.43: Effect of laser vision correction on spherical aberration.

converts the cornea into oblate and induces more +ve SA, as shown in **Figure 2.43**.

Studying corneal wavefront is important for the following reasons:

- Explain the symptoms of the patient. Patients with abnormal HOAs may suffer from glare, halos, ghost images, shadows, or starbursts.

- Explain the suboptimal corrected visual acuity. When the HOAs are significant, the quality and quantity of vision are suboptimal.
- HOAs can be used to distinguish early keratoconus from normal and to grade the severity of keratoconus.
- Select the best laser profile in laser-based refractive surgery. When the HOAs are abnormal and symptomatic, customized rather than optimized laser vision correction is indicated.
- Select the best type of intraocular lens in lens-based refractive surgery and cataract by following the Practical Subjective IOL Selection (PSIS) algorithm.

THE PRACTICAL SUBJECTIVE IOL SELECTION (PSIS) ALGORITHM

The PSIS algorithm helps the surgeon in selecting the IOL type that best suits the eye based on three factors:
1. Patient's demands (depth of focus vs. quality of the vision).
2. The RMS of HOAs.
3. The ZC of the SA.

The PSIS algorithm is applied in lens-based refractive surgery, particularly clear lens extraction (Chapter 5), and cataract surgery (Chapter 6).

There are general guidelines that rule the PSIS algorithm:
1. If DOF is critical to the patient, maintain or shift the SA to the non-toxic zone as much as possible.
2. If the image quality is critical to the patient, target $+0.1\ \mu m$ of SA as much as possible. It has been found that when the ocular SA $= +0.1\ \mu m$, visual acuity is optimum.
3. Premium IOLs (multifocal, trifocal, EDOF) are possible when the total RMS is $\leq 0.35\ \mu m$.

4. There are three types of IOLs in terms of IOL asphericity and SA:

   (a) The traditional spheric IOL, which generates +ve SA.

   (b) The zero-SA aspheric IOL, which is a parabolic aspheric IOL generating no SA.

   (c) The –ve SA aspheric IOL, which is an aspheric IOL generating –ve SA. Currently, there are two types of the –ve SA IOLs: the one that generates –0.20 µm of SA, and the one that generates –0.27 µm of SA.

Figures 2.44 to 2.47 illustrate the PSIS algorithm.

A. The total RMS ≤0.35 µm **(Fig. 2.44)**:

   1. *The DOF is critical to the patient:* Premium IOL implantation is possible (See Chapter 5).

   2. *The image quality is critical to the patient:* Use a monofocal IOL that compensates for the corneal SA.

      a. If the SA is ≥ +0.2 µm, select an aspheric IOL with –ve SA to achieve a residual SA = +0.1 µm.

      b. If the SA is around +0.1 µm, use an aspheric IOL with zero-SA.

B. The total RMS >±0.35 µm on account of HOAs rather than the SA **(Fig. 2.44)**: Use an aspheric IOL with zero-SA to avoid complicating the HOAs.

C. The total RMS >±0.35 µm on account of the SA:

   1. The patient has a previous hyperopic laser treatment (the cornea has -ve SA) **(Fig. 2.45)**:

      a. The –ve SA is non-toxic:

         • The DOF is critical to the patient, use an aspheric IOL with zero-SA to maintain the –ve non-toxic SA and the DOF that the cornea has.

         • The image quality is critical to the patient, use a spheric IOL (+ve SA by default) to compensate for the -ve SA that the cornea has.

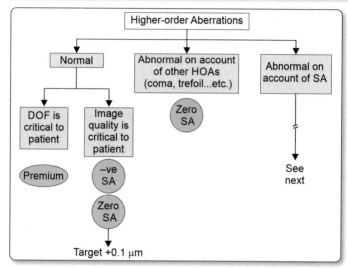

Fig. 2.44: The Practical Subjective IOL Selection (PSIS) algorithm in normal and abnormal higher-order aberrations.

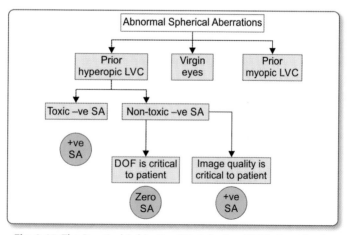

Fig. 2.45: The Practical Subjective IOL Selection (PSIS) algorithm in post-hyperopic laser vision correction (LVC).

    b. The –ve SA is toxic, use a spheric IOL (+ve SA by default) to reduce the toxic –ve SA and shift it as close to the non-toxic –ve SA as possible.

2. The patient has a previous myopic laser treatment (+ve SA) **(Fig. 2.46)**:

    a. *The +ve SA is non-toxic:*

- The DOF is critical to the patient, use an aspheric IOL with zero-SA to maintain the +ve non-toxic SA and the DOF that the cornea has.
- The image quality is critical to the patient, select an aspheric IOL with –0.27 µm SA to reduce the non-toxic SA as much as possible.

    b. *The SA is toxic:* Select the aspheric IOL with –0.27 µm SA to reduce the toxic +ve SA as much as possible and convert it into non-toxic if possible.

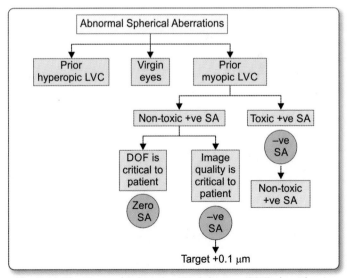

Fig. 2.46: The Practical Subjective IOL Selection (PSIS) algorithm in post-myopic laser vision correction (LVC).

3. The eye is virgin (non-operated) **(Fig. 2.47)**:
    a. *The +ve SA is non-toxic:*
        - The DOF is critical to the patient, use an aspheric IOL with zero-SA to maintain the non-toxic +ve SA and the DOF that the cornea has.
        - The image quality is critical to the patient, select the aspheric IOL with –0.27 μm SA to reduce the non-toxic SA as much as possible.
    b. *The +ve SA is toxic:* This is a rare condition. Select the aspheric IOL with –0.27 μm SA to reduce the toxic SA as much as possible and convert it into non-toxic if possible.

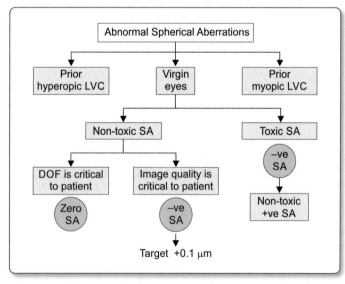

Fig. 2.47: The Practical Subjective IOL Selection (PSIS) algorithm in virgin non-operated cornea.

■ REGULARITY VERSUS RISK SCORING

It is essential to differentiate between being an irregular cornea and being a cornea at risk based on the PS3. The cornea may be regular but at high risk and may be irregular but still within the low-risk range. For example, it is not uncommon to encounter keratoconus with a symmetric bowtie on the anterior curvature map. On the other hand, low-risk corneas may have some irregularities. **Figure 2.48** represents a low-risk curvature map as per PS3 because S-I < 2.5 D. However, because the superior part is steeper than the inferior part, the RMS is high, particularly the coma, as shown in **Figure 2.49**.

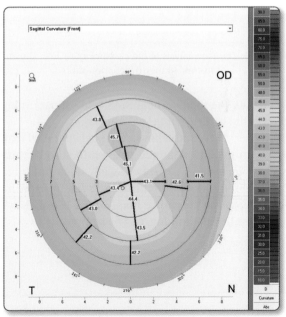

Fig. 2.48: The anterior sagittal curvature map at low-risk.

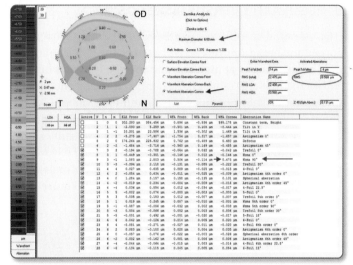

Fig. 2.49: Zernike analysis of the case in Figure 2.48, showing abnormal higher-order aberrations.

In this figure, the total corneal RMS (red eclipse) is high on account of the vertical coma (red arrows).

Moreover, the introduction of corneal epithelial mapping into screening has changed the understanding of risk factors. Unfortunately, the Pentacam does not have this kind of mapping. However, it is interesting to know that an asymmetry on the curvature map, which is not associated with focal epithelial thinning, can be ignored.

Exclude Ectatic Corneal Diseases: Tomographic Characteristics of Ectatic Corneal Diseases

Ectatic corneal diseases (ECDs) are the main source of irregular astigmatism. They can be categorized into:

- *Established ectasia:* Keratoconus (KC), Pellucid Marginal Degeneration (PMD), Pellucid-Like Keratoconus (PLK), Keratoglobus (KG) and Postlaser vision correction (post-LVC) ectasia.
- *Para ectasia:* Forme Fruste Keratoconus (FFKC) and Keratoconus Suspect (KCS).
- *Corneas with high potential:* Posterior keratoconus, apparently normal corneas, and unclassified abnormal corneas.

■ TOMOGRAPHIC DEFINITION OF ECDs

Established Ectasia or ECDs Per Se

- *Keratoconus (KC):* It is characterized by a combination of an abnormal anterior curvature map and an abnormal posterior elevation map. That is regardless of the pachymetry map as KC may be encountered in thick corneas **(Fig. 3.1)**, while thin corneas may be normal **(Fig. 3.2)**.
- *Pellucid Marginal Degeneration (PMD) (Fig. 3.3):* It is described by a combination of a crab-claw pattern on the anterior curvature map and an abnormal posterior elevation map. Since the crab-claw pattern is not diagnostic of PMD, the "Bell sign" on the pachymetry map is the hallmark of PMD that differentiates it from Pellucid-Like Keratoconus (PLK).

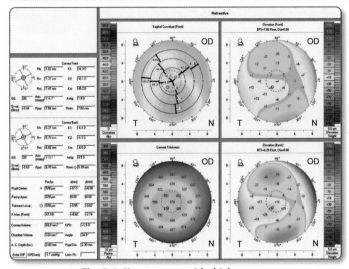

Fig. 3.1: Keratoconus with thick cornea.

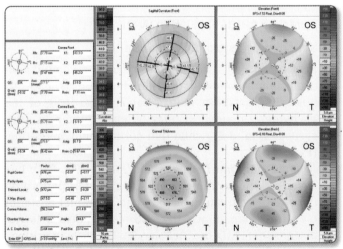

Fig. 3.2: Normal thin cornea.

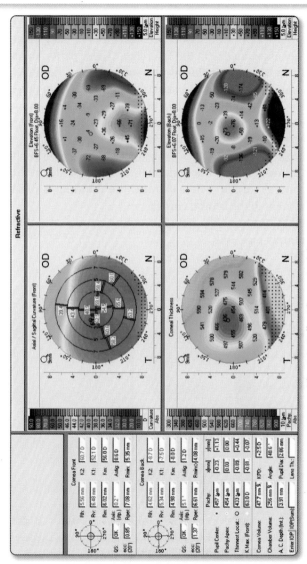

Fig. 3.3: Pellucid marginal degeneration.

- *Pellucid-Like Keratoconus (PLK)* **(Fig. 3.4):** There are patterns of KC that are associated with the crab-claw shape but not associated with the "Bell sign." These patterns can be given the term "Pellucid-Like Keratoconus" or "PLK." In some cases, PLK can be an early stage of PMD. In other words, if PLK is diagnosed, it should be monitored as it may convert into PMD, especially if the pachymetry map shows the "droplet" sign (*see* **Fig. 2.15**).
- *Keratoglobus (KG)* **(Fig. 3.5):** The cornea in KG is diffusely steep, and diffusely thinned, often more markedly in the peripheral cornea, whereas in KC the thinning is most prominent in the central cornea.
- *Post-LVC Ectasia* **(Fig. 3.6):** It usually occurs post-LASIK and rarely post-PRK. It may take the pattern of KC, PLK, or PMD.

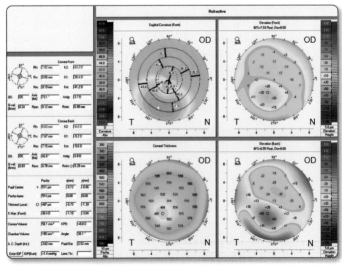

Fig. 3.4: Pellucid-like keratoconus.

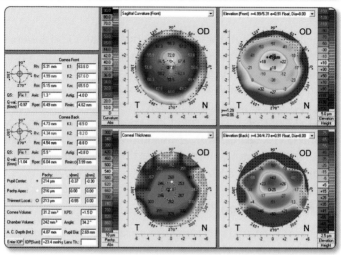

Fig. 3.5: Keratoglobus.

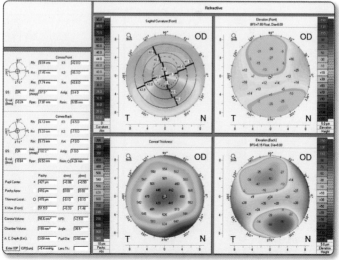

Fig. 3.6: Post laser vision correction ectasia.

Para Ectasia

It includes Forme Fruste Keratoconus (FFKC) and Keratoconus Suspect (KCS). These two terms describe the same abnormality, which is characterized by an abnormal anterior curvature map and a normal posterior elevation map **(Fig. 3.7)**. When this abnormality is in one eye while the other eye has KC (or any other ECD per se), this abnormality is called FFKC **(Fig. 3.8)**. If this abnormality is in one eye while the other eye is normal or has the same abnormality, it is called KCS **(Fig. 3.9)**.

Corneas with High Potential

This entity consists of posterior keratoconus, apparently normal corneas, and unclassified abnormal corneas.

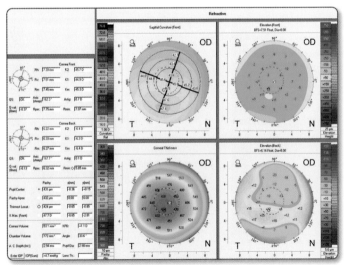

Fig. 3.7: Para ectasia.

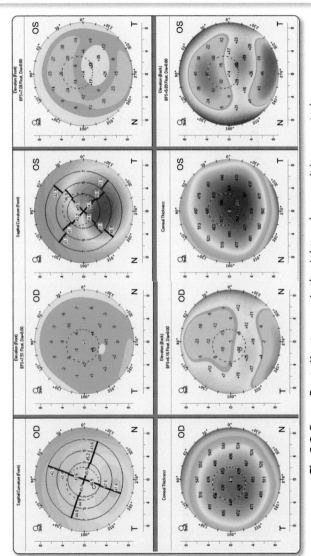

Fig. 3.8: Forme Fruste Keratoconus in the right eye because it is para ectasia, and the other eye has keratoconus.

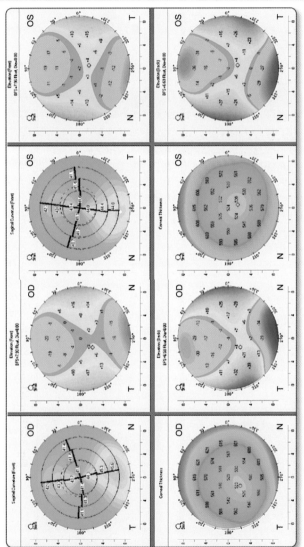

Fig. 3.9: Keratoconus suspect in both eyes because it is para ectasia in both eyes.

- *Posterior keratoconus:* It is characterized by a normal anterior curvature map and an abnormal posterior elevation map **(Fig. 3.10)**.
- *Apparently normal corneas:* It is the case of bilateral tomographically normal corneas with a positive family history of an ECD.
- *Unclassified abnormal corneas:* They are corneas that demonstrate abnormalities that are significantly outside the normal range but do not meet the criteria of ECDs. This term describes the corneas that have one high risk or two moderate risk factors in the Practical Subjective Scoring System (PS3) *and are not* categorized under any of the previous entities.

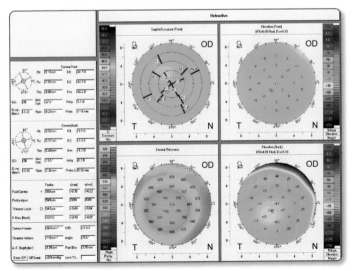

Fig. 3.10: Posterior keratoconus.

■ PROGRESSION CRITERIA

Defining progression of the ECDs is a necessity for both indication of treatment, particularly corneal crosslinking (CXL), and the follow-up after treatment to observe efficacy and failure. The best method to observe progression is the Belin "ABCD" Keratoconus Staging. If it is not available, the maximum K-readings (Kmax) AND thinnest corneal thickness (TCT) can roughly be used.

Belin "ABCD" Keratoconus Staging

This grading system depends on observing the changes in four parameters (**Fig. 3.11**), the radii of curvature of the anterior (A) and posterior (B) surfaces of a 3-mm area around the thinnest location, thickness (C) of the thinnest location, and distance corrected visual acuity (D). There are two displays of this staging, the individual one per visit, as shown in **Figure 3.11**, and the comparative one that compares between visits and displays the changes. **Figure 3.12** is an example of three visits of follow-up. The first-visit bars are colored in orange, the second-visit bars are colored in green, and the third-visit bars are colored in brown. As shown in the top of the figure, the dotted green line represents 80% of confidence interval (CI) Normal, the solid green line represents 95% CI Normal, the dotted red line represents 80% CI KC (or any ECD per se), and the solid red line represents 95% CI KC (or any ECD per se). The first visit is usually used as a baseline exam (BE) for comparisons (red arrow). According to Michael Belin, a jump of one parameter beyond the 95% CI normal or two parameters beyond the 80% CI normal is considered as progression. The intervals between the visits should be at least 3 months. In **Figure 3.12**, the A and B parameters

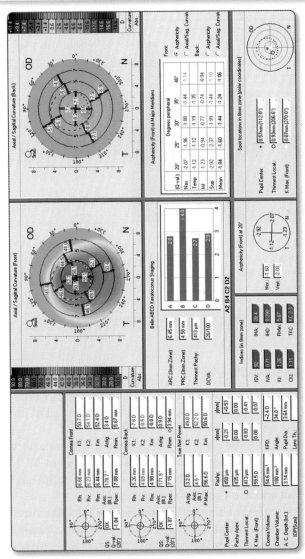

Fig. 3.11: Belin "ABCD" Keratoconus Staging. The individual display per visit.

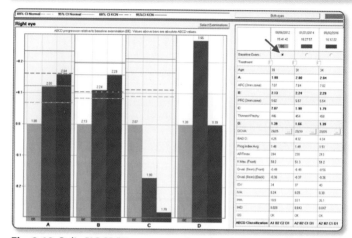

Fig. 3.12: Belin "ABCD" Keratoconus Staging. The comparative display. The red arrow indicates the baseline exam (BE) to which the sequential exams are compared.

jumped beyond the 80% line in the next visit in comparison with the BE, and both of them reached beyond the 95% in the third visit.

Parametric Progression

If the ABCD software is not available, maximum K-reading (Kmax) and TCT are to be observed. The following steps are recommended:

1. Take at least three captures per cornea per visit and check the quality of the captures, as mentioned in Chapter 1.
2. The three captures better be taken by the same technician per visit and in every visit if possible.
3. Compare the medians. The median Kmax of the three captures in a visit is compared with the median Kmax of the three captures in the next visit.

4. Along the observation period (usually 3 to 6 months), an increase in Kmax $\geq$ 1.5 D *and* a thinning in the TCT $\geq$ 15 µm is considered a progression. Please note that both parameters should change to consider that a progression. If only one parameter changes, it is an artifact.

■ TO CROSSLINK OR NOT TO CROSSLINK

- In the case of KC and PLK, the cutoff age beyond which they are considered stable is still debatable and subject to population. In some populations, KC and PLK may progress until the age of 30 years. In general, if the age is below 25 years, CXL is indicated.
- PMD is progressive whatever the age is, therefore CXL is indicated.
- KG is usually not progressive or minimally progressive. However, in the absence of a definitive standard procedure for the management of this disorder, it deserves to be crosslinked because it is thin and fragile, especially since new CXL protocols are recently available for ultra-thin corneas.
- Post-LVC ectasia is always progressive and should be crosslinked urgently.
- Both KCS and FFKC should be observed. In the case of progression, CXL is indicated.
- If posterior keratoconus is bilateral and symmetric, it is a congenital malformation rather than an ectasia, but should be monitored. If the case is unilateral or asymmetric, it is most probably a developing ectasia, i.e., prestage of KC, and action should be taken. For example, if a child has asymmetric posterior keratoconus, CXL should be performed.

- In apparently normal corneas with a strong family history, CXL is *not* indicated.
- In unclassified abnormal corneas, CXL is *not* indicated.

■ OBSERVATION AFTER CORNEAL CROSSLINKING

As soon as CXL has been performed, the cornea starts to change. Two major changes are encountered, steepening and thinning. K-readings usually increase from the preoperative baseline by 2–3 D during the first 3 months **(Fig. 3.13)**. After that, they decrease back to the baseline during the second 3 months. Subsequently, they keep decreasing by an additional 2–3 D over the following 2 years. Steepening during the first 3 months is associated with thinning of the cornea; the cornea loses about 30–50 μm of its thickness **(Fig. 3.14)**. However, the cornea starts retrieving its original thickness

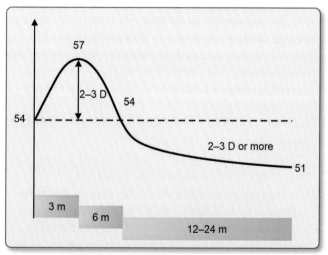

Fig. 3.13: Changes in K-readings after corneal crosslinking.

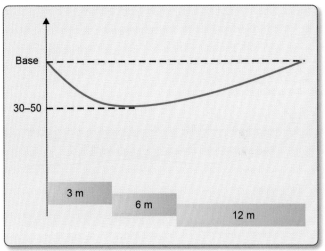

Fig. 3.14: Changes in corneal thickness after corneal crosslinking.

during the second 3 months and usually reaches the preoperative baseline thickness almost 12 months after CXL.

In conclusion, during the first 6 months, it is incorrect to observe the progression of ECDs, and therefore the failure of CXL because the changes produced by the CXL during the first 6 months are very similar to the progression of the disease **(Fig. 3.15)**.

◼ ENTITIES MISDIAGNOSED AS ECTASIA (EMEs)

Any corneal irregularities can be misdiagnosed as ECDs. EMEs result from factors of false findings, especially previous corneal surgeries (e.g., LASIK, PRK, SMILE, RK, corneal graft, etc.) and corneal opacities. Therefore, it is essential to follow the definition of ECDs and to classify the patterns of other

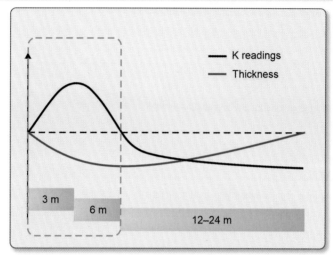

Fig. 3.15: Changes in K-readings and corneal thickness after corneal crosslinking. The changes during the first 6 months are similar to disease progression.

corneal irregularities into three patterns, contour, hot spot, and discrete patterns. The most useful maps to study the patterns and differentiate them from ECDs are the anterior tangential map and the relative pachymetry map.

Best Maps for Diagnosis

- *The anterior tangential map:* It is the best curvature map to describe the geography of irregularities and to show the real efficient postoperative optical zone, as shown in **Figure 3.16**. It is less affected by misalignment, but it overestimates K-readings.
- *The relative pachymetry map:* It helps to identify the ablated corneal zones. The map takes disciform, donut, or elongated shapes after myopic, hyperopic, or astigmatic ablations, respectively. If the zone of high negative values

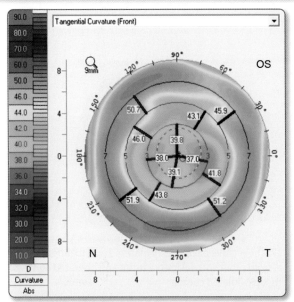

Fig. 3.16: The anterior tangential curvature map as a tool to differentiate ectatic diseases from other corneal irregularities and operated corneas. It describes the contour effect. This is a case of post myopic ablated cornea.

is central **(Fig. 3.17)**, the ablation was central (myopic treatment). If the zone of negative values is peripheral **(Fig. 3.18)**, the ablation was peripheral (hyperopic treatment). If the zone of negative values is elongated, the ablation was astigmatic **(Fig. 3.19)**.

Patterns of Corneal Irregularities

Contour Pattern

The contour pattern usually takes the shape of a ring or a zone, describing the junction between two different corneal zones, the zone of treatment and the untreated corneal zone.

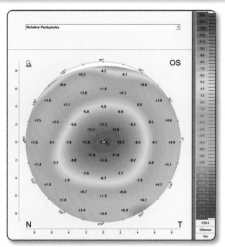

Fig. 3.17: The relative pachymetry map as a tool to differentiate ectatic diseases from other corneal irregularities and operated corneas. This is a post myopic ablated cornea.

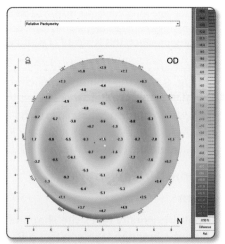

Fig. 3.18: Post hyperopic ablated cornea.

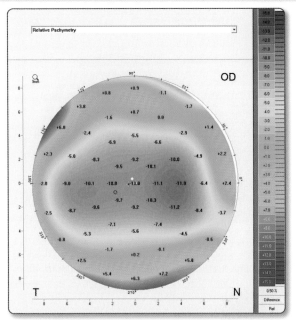

Fig. 3.19: Post astigmatic ablated cornea.

These patterns are seen after LVC (*see* **Fig. 3.16**), corneal grafts **(Fig. 3.20)**, and after intracorneal rings (ICRs) implantation **(Fig. 3.21)**. In the case of a decentered optical zone after LVC **(Fig. 3.22)**, it can be confused with post-LVC ectasia. Contrary to post-LVC ectasia, the contour area is not associated with correspondent thinning and posterior elevation steepening.

Hot Spot Pattern

This pattern results from contact lenses, tear film disturbance, *focal* corneal opacities and pathologies, and inadequate exposure to the camera.

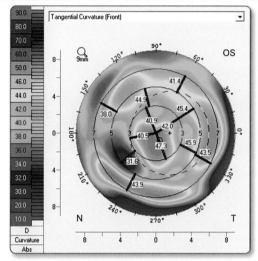

Fig. 3.20: Contour effect post corneal graft.

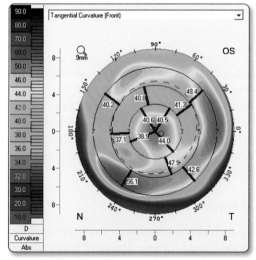

Fig. 3.21: Contour effect after intracorneal ring implantation.

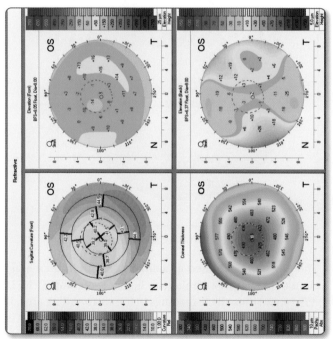

Fig. 3.22: Contour effect in decentered ablation zone.

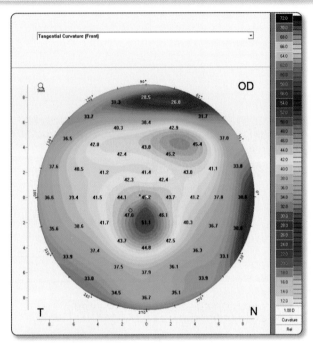

Fig. 3.23: The hot spot pattern.

The hot spot is defined as a small (≤3 mm in diameter) circular or oval area of relatively higher K-readings (≥1.5 D difference) than the K-readings in the surrounding area. It can be located in any sector of the cornea. **Figure 3.23** is an example of this pattern.

Discrete Pattern

It results from tear film disturbance, *multifocal* corneal opacities and pathologies, corneal grafts, and inadequate exposure to the camera. **Figure 3.24** is an example of this pattern.

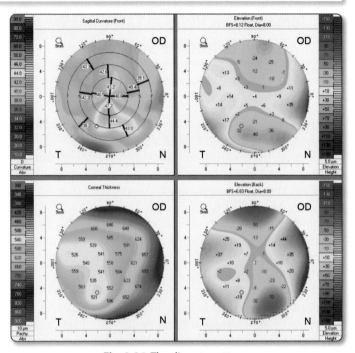

Fig. 3.24: The discrete pattern.

Tomographic Rules in Laser-based Refractive Surgery

This type is cornea-based. Subtypes can be categorized into surface photoablation and lamellar photoablation.

Surface photoablation consists of Photorefractive Keratectomy (PRK), Laser Subepithelial Keratomileusis (LASEK), Epipolis Laser in Situ Keratomileusis (Epi-LASIK), and Trans-Epithelial Photorefractive Keratectomy (TE-PRK).

Lamellar photoablation consists of Laser in Situ Keratomileusis (LASIK), Femtosecond Laser in Situ Keratomileusis (FemtoLASIK), sub-Bowman Keratomileusis (SBK), and Small Incision Lenticule Extraction (SMILE).

The subtypes of laser-based refractive surgery have rules in common and rules in specific. The rules in common are rules of K-readings, optical zone (OZ), cyclotorsion, recentration of the laser profile, and astigmatic disparity. The rules in specific are the thickness rules.

▪ RULES OF REFRACTIVE ERROR MAGNITUDE

Table 4.1 shows the recommended range of correction of refractive error magnitude for surface ablation and LASIK. It is highly recommended to avoid corrections beyond the limits to avoid complications even if other rules allow for the correction. **Table 4.2** represents six examples.

Regarding the SMILE, there are two schools differing in the pre- and intraoperative treatment parameters. **Table 4.3** shows the parameters in the European CE Mark and the FDA Approval. **Table 4.4** represents six examples.

Table 4.1: Range of refractive error magnitude to be treated.

	Myopic SE (D)	Hypermetropic SE (D)	Astigmatism (D)
Surface Ablation	Up to −8.00	Not recommended	Up to 2.00[a]
LASIK	Up to −8.00	Up to +6.00	Up to 6.00

(SE: spherical equivalent)
[a]Not recommended above 2.00 D because of the epithelial remodeling effect.

Table 4.2: Examples of range of refractive error magnitude.

Example	Sphere (D)	Cylinder (D)	SE (D)	Surface Ablation	LASIK
1	−4.00	−2.00	−5.00	✓	✓
2	−7.00	−3.50	−8.75	X	X
3	+3.00	+1.50	+3.75	X	✓
4	−9.00	0	−9.00	X	X
5	−2.50	−5.00	−5.00	X	✓
6	+2.50	−4.00	+0.50	X	✓

(SE: spherical equivalent)

Table 4.3: Parameters of SMILE treatment in CE mark and FDA approval.

Parameter	CE Mark	2018 FDA Approval
Sphere to be treated	−0.50 to −10.00 D	−1.00 to −10.00 D
Preoperative cylinder	No restriction	Up to −3.00 D
Cylinder to be treated	Up to −5.00 D	−0.50 to −3.00 D
SE to be treated	−0.50 to −12.50 D	−1.00 to −11.50 D
Preoperative SE	No restriction	Up to −11.50 D

(SE: spherical equivalent; SMILE: small incision lenticule extraction)

Table 4.4: Examples of selection criteria in SMILE based on refraction.

| Example | Preoperative Refraction | | | Treatment Plan | | | CE Mark | 2018 FDA Approval |
	Sphere (D)	Cylinder (D)	SE (D)	Sphere (D)	Cylinder (D)	SE (D)		
1	−3.00	−2.00	−4.00	Full correction			✓	✓
2	−6.00	−1.00	−6.50	Full correction			✓	✓
3	−11.00	−5.00	−13.50	−10.00	−3.00	−11.50	✓	✗
4	−5.00	−4.00	−7.00	Full correction			✓	✗
5	−10.00	−4.00	−12.00	−9.00	−2.50	−10.25	✓	✗
6	−12.50	−3.00	−14.00	Full correction			✗	✗

(SE: spherical equivalent)

■ THICKNESS RULES

Total refraction (TR) and central ablation depth (CAD) are used for thickness calculations.

1. *Calculating TR:* TR is the algebraic sum of the sphere and cylinder. **Table 4.5** represents six examples.
2. *Calculating CAD:* CAD depends on the magnitude and the type of the corrected refractive error, optical (OZ), and treated (TZ) zones, laser profile (optimized versus customized). In customized laser profiles, CAD can only be calculated by the machine software. Therefore, all calculations in this book will be based on the optimized laser profiles.

   In optimized laser profiles, CAD is calculated by Munnerlyn formula:

   $CAD = 1/3 \times (OZ \text{ in mm})^2 \times$ intended correction in dioptres, where the intended correction is the TR in most softwares. To make the calculations more practical, follow **Table 4.6**. **Table 4.7** represents six examples.
3. *Thickness rules in surface ablation:*
   A. Preoperatively, CCT should be ≥470 μm (including the epithelium).
   B. Postoperatively, CCT should be ≥400 μm (including the epithelium).

Example	Sphere (D)	Cylinder (D)	TR (D)
1	−2.00	−4.00	−6.00
2	−3.00	−1.00	−4.00
3	+4.00	−1.50	+2.50
4	+5.00	+1.00	+6.00
5	+2.00	−3.00	−1.00
6	+2.00	−4.00	−2.00

Table 4.5: Examples of total refraction (TR).

Table 4.6: Central ablation depth (CAD).

		OZ		
	TR	6.00 mm	6.50 mm	7.00 mm
CAD	Per −1.00 D	13 μm	15 μm	17 μm
	Per +1.00 D	0 μm	0 μm	0 μm

(TR: total refraction; OZ: optical zone)

Table 4.7: Examples of central ablation depth (CAD).

				CAD (μm)		
Examples	Sphere (D)	Cylinder (D)	TR (D)	OZ = 6.00 mm	OZ = 6.50 mm	OZ = 7.00 mm
1	−2.00	−4.00	−6.00	78	90	102
2	−3.00	−1.00	−4.00	52	60	68
3	+4.00	−1.50	+2.50	0	0	0
4	+5.00	+1.00	+6.00	0	0	0
5	+2.00	−3.00	−1.00	13	15	17
6	+2.00	−4.00	−2.00	26	30	34

(TR: total refraction; OZ: optical zone)

The postoperative corneal thickness after surface ablation is calculated as follows:

Postoperative CCT (including epithelium) = Preoperative CCT (including epithelium) − CAD

Table 4.8 shows six examples.

4. *Thickness rules in LASIK and FemtoLASIK:*

   A. Preoperatively, CCT should be ≥500 μm (including the epithelium).

   B. Postoperatively, Percent Tissue Altered (PTA) <40%.

   PTA takes into consideration flap thickness (FT), CAD, and CCT. It is calculated by the formula:

   $$PTA = (FT + CAD) \times 100/CCT$$

Table 4.8: Examples of thickness rules in surface ablation.

Examples	TR (D)	CAD (μm) OZ = 6.50 mm	Preoperative CCT (μm)	Postoperative CCT (μm)	Surface Ablation
1	−8.00	120	480	360	X
2	−5.00	75	515	440	✓
3	+3.50	0	470	470	✓
4	+5.00	0	517	517	✓
5	−1.50	22.5	495	472.5	✓
6	−6.00	90	485	395	X

(TR: total refraction; CAD: central ablation depth; OZ: optical zone; CCT: central corneal thickness)

The normal PTA is <40%. **Table 4.9** represents six examples.

5. *Thickness rules in SMILE:* **Figures 4.1 and 4.2** illustrate SMILE components. As shown in these figures, the lenticule is composed between the cap (superior) cut and the refractive (inferior) cut, and it is extracted through the small side incision (the entrance incision). The corneal above the lenticule, including the epithelium, is called "the cap," and below the lenticule is called "the bed."

In terms of thickness rules, the following rules are recommended:

A. Preoperatively, CCT should be ≥470 μm (including the epithelium).

B. *Intraoperatively:*

   i. *Cap thickness:* The recommended cap thickness ranges from 120 μm to 135 μm. The latter is preferable because it helps for future enhancement. If FemtoLASIK is planned for enhancement, a 100-μm flap will be safe enough to avoid interference with the epithelium above

Table 4.9: Examples of percent tissue altered (PTA).

Examples	TR (D)	CAD (μm) OZ = 6.5 mm	Pre-op CCT (μm)	Flap = 130 (μm)	Flap = 120 (μm)	Flap = 110 (μm)	Flap = 100 (μm)	Flap = 90 (μm)	LASIK and FemtoLASIK
						PTA (%)			
1	−9.00	135	530	50	48.1	46.2	44.3	42.5	x
2	−6.00	90	520	42.3	40.4	38.5	36.5	34.6	✓ (Flap ≤110 μm)
3	+2.50	0	480	27.1	25	22.9	20.8	18.8	x
4	+6.00	0	512	25.4	23.4	21.5	19.5	17.6	✓
5	−1.00	15	487	29.8	27.7	25.7	23.6	21.6	x
6	−2.00	30	532	30.1	28.2	26.3	24.4	22.6	✓

(TR: total refraction; CAD: central ablation depth; OZ: optical zone; CCT: central corneal thickness; PTA: percent tissue altered)

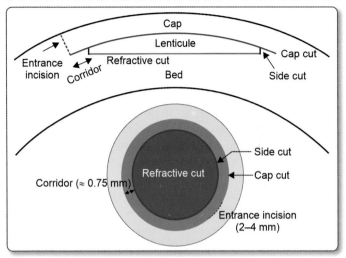

Fig. 4.1: Components of the small incision lenticule extraction (SMILE).

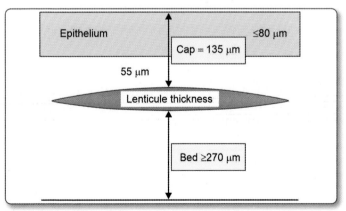

Fig. 4.2: Illustration of the small incision lenticule extraction (SMILE) showing the epithelium layer (≤80 μm), the recommended cap thickness (135 μm), and the recommended bed thickness (≥270 μm). These recommendations allow for future enhancement by LASIK and PRK.

and the previous cap cut below. If PRK is planned for enhancement, the 55-μm stroma above the cap should be sufficient.

  ii. *Side cut:* The myopic lenticule does not taper to 0 thickness at its edge. The edge is known as the side cut. The surgeon can choose the thickness of the side cut to be 10–30 μm. Most surgeons choose 15 μm. However, the thickness can be reduced to 10 μm in high myopic corrections (e.g., –10.00), and can be increased to 20–25 μm in low myopic corrections (e.g., –2.00).

  iii. *Bed thickness:* The minimum should range between 250 and 280 μm. The latter is more preferable.

C. Postoperatively, CCT should be ≥400 μm (including the epithelium).

Table 4.10 represents six examples assuming that cap thickness is 135 μm and side cut thickness is 15 μm. These examples were calculated by using SMILE software.

Table 4.10: Examples of thickness rules in SMILE (Cap = 135 μm; Side = 15 μm).

Examples	TR (D)	Preoperative CCT (μm)	OZ (mm)	Lenticule Thickness (μm)	Bed Thickness (μm)	Postoperative CCT (μm)	SMILE
1	–8.00	550	6.5	135	280	415	✓
2	–5.00	515	6.5	93	287	422	✓
3	–3.50	495	7	82	278	413	✓
4	–10.00	520	6.5	161	224	359	X
5	–12.00	560	6.5	188	237	372	X
6	–6.75	545	7	137	273	408	✓

(TR: total refraction; CCT: central corneal thickness; OZ: optical zone)

Table 4.11: Examples of thickness rules in SMILE (Cap = 120 µm; Side = 10 µm).

Examples	TR (D)	Preoperative CCT (µm)	Optical Zone (mm)	Lenticule Thickness (µm)	Bed Thickness (µm)	Postoperative CCT (µm)	SMILE
1	–8.00	550	6.5	135	300	415	✓
2	–5.00	515	6.5	93	307	422	✓
3	–3.50	495	7	82	318	413	✓
4	–10.00	520	6.5	161	244	359	X
5	–12.00	560	6.5	188	257	372	✓
6	–6.75	545	7	137	273	408	✓

(TR: total refraction; CCT: central corneal thickness; OZ: optical zone)

Table 4.11 represents the same examples in **Table 4.10**, but assuming that cap thickness is 120 µm and side cut thickness is 10 µm. These examples were calculated by using SMILE software.

■ K-READINGS RULES

The spherical equivalent (SE) is used in K-reading calculations. It affects the mean anterior K-reading (Km).

1. *Calculating the SE:* SE is calculated by the formula:

$$SE = Sphere + (Cylinder/2)$$

Table 4.12 represents six examples.

2. Calculating the predicted postoperative K-readings. In general, every –1 D SE correction reduces Km by 0.8 D, and every + 1 D SE correction increases Km by 1.25 D. Whatever the type of the refractive error, the SE is applied on the preoperative Km to predict the postoperative Km.

The postoperative Km should remain in the range of 34–49 D. Going below 34 D or above 49 D carries the risk of toxic (intolerable) spherical aberrations. **Table 4.13** shows six examples.

Table 4.12: Examples of spherical equivalent (SE) calculation.			
Example	Sphere (D)	Cylinder (D)	SE (D)
1	–2.00	–4.00	–4.00
2	–3.00	–1.00	–3.50
3	+4.00	–1.50	+3.25
4	+5.00	+1.00	+5.50
5	+2.00	–3.00	+0.50
6	+2.00	–4.00	0

(SE: spherical equivalent)

Table 4.13: Examples of changes in anterior mean K-reading (Km).					
Examples	SE (D)	Changes in Km (D)	Pre-op Km (D)	Post-op Km (D)	Corneal Refractive Surgeries
1	–9.00	–9.00 × 0.80 = –7.2	40	32.8	X
2	–4.50	–4.50 × 0.80 = –3.6	44.5	40.9	✓
3	+3.50	+3.50 × 1.25 = +4.38	46	50.38	X
4	+4.50	+4.50 × 1.25 = +5.63	42	47.63	✓
5	0	0	47.08	47.08	✓
6	–3.75	–3.75 × 0.80 = –3.00	41.05	37.05	✓

(SE: spherical aberration; Km: mean K-reading on anterior surface)

■ OPTICAL ZONE (OZ) AND MESOPIC PUPIL RULES

- If preoperative mesopic pupil is >7 mm, laser-based refractive surgery is contraindicated.
- If preoperative mesopic pupil is <2 mm or >6 mm, premium lens implantation is contraindicated.
- In laser-based refractive surgery, the OZ should equal mesopic pupil + 0.5 mm.
- In myopic ablation, the OZ should be ≥6 mm.
- In hyperopic ablation, the OZ should be ≥7 mm.
- In high ablations (high refractive errors), reducing the OZ to gain more tissue and, therefore, more corrected diopters, makes the efficient OZ (the actual achieved postoperative OZ shown by the tangential map) less than what was attempted to be. Therefore, it is strongly recommended not to reduce the OZ, especially in high corrections, to avoid induction of spherical aberration.

Table 4.14 shows six examples.

Table 4.14: Examples of optical zone and mesopic pupil rules in laser-based refractive surgery.

Examples	SE (D)	Mesopic Pupil (mm)	OZ (mm)	Surface Ablation
1	−5.00	6.00	6.5	✓
2	−4.50	6.10	6.6	✓
3	0	5.20	6	✓
4	+4.50	7.10	7.6	X
5	+1.50	3.70	7	✓
6	−2.75	5.70	6.2	✓

(SE: spherical aberration; OZ: optical zone)

■ CYCLOTORSION RULES

In astigmatic correction, the laser profile should exactly match where it should be applied on the cornea. The eyes usually experience cyclotorsion when changing the position from the sitting position (status of capturing tomography) to the supine position (status of operation). This cyclotorsion affects astigmatic correction. In case of mismatch, the angle of error causes resultant residual astigmatism, which has a different axis and is irregular in many cases. There is a proportional relationship between the angle of error and the magnitude of the residual astigmatism, and between the latter and the magnitude of the pre-operative astigmatism. **Figure 4.3** shows the proportional relationship between the angle of error and the magnitude of the residual astigmatism. If the angle of error was 10°, the magnitude of the resultant astigmatism equals

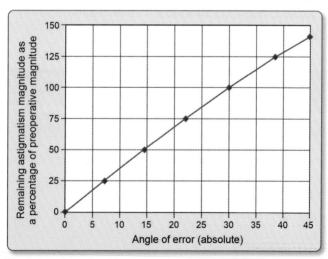

Fig. 4.3: Cyclotorsion. The proportional relationship between angle of error and the magnitude of the resultant residual astigmatism.

a third of the preoperative astigmatism but on a different axis. For example, if the preoperative astigmatism was 4.50 D, the resultant astigmatism is 1.50 D on a new axis. Cyclotorsion usually has a significant impact when the magnitude of the planned astigmatic correction is ≥1.50 D.

■ RECENTRATION RULES

The eye uses the visual axis rather than the pupil axis when looking at an object. All excimer laser machines are programmed to recognize the pupil center to center the laser profiles. To obtain perfect visual performance and avoid induction of higher-order aberrations (HOAs), particularly coma, the laser profiles should be centered on the visual axis. This can be achieved by the recentration technique, which differs from a machine to another. Recentration is important when angle kappa is >200 μm and:

- The myopic astigmatism is >1.50 D.
- In case of any hyperopic refractive errors, such as hyperopia, hyperopic astigmatism, and mixed astigmatism.

Recentration includes two elements, centering the laser profile by the magnitude of angle kappa, and centering the flap on the visual axis (first Purkinje). In addition, in the case of any hyperopic element, the flap size should be adjusted to avoid any out-of-the-bed ablation. The technique is discussed in the "Five Steps To Start Your Refractive Surgery" book.

■ RULES OF HIGHER ORDER ABERRATIONS (HOAs)

As mentioned in Chapter 2, the total RMS of corneal HOAs is normally ≤0.35 μm (≤0.50 D). The higher the RMS, the more severe the irregularity.

- If the corneal HOAs RMS is abnormal and the patient has symptoms such as glare and halos (spherical aberration), ghost images and shadows (coma), or starbursts (trefoil), customized laser vision correction (LVC) rather than the traditional LVC is recommended.

- If the corneal HOAs RMS is abnormal, but the patient has no symptoms, it is highly recommended to avoid customized LVC because such HOAs either are native and do not affect the patient or are compensated for by the crystalline lens. In both cases, no need to interfere with them; otherwise, the patient suffers from postoperative new iatrogenic HOAs that may or may not be compensated for by neural adaptation.

■ RULES OF ASTIGMATIC DISPARITY

As described in Chapter 1, a difference between tomographic astigmatism (TA) and subjective manifest astigmatism (MA) of ≥1.00 D in magnitude or ≥10° in axis is considered abnormal, and the capture should be repeated. If the disparity continues to appear in the following captures, specific causes should be inspected. **Table 4.15** shows six examples of the astigmatic disparity.

Table 4.15: Examples of astigmatic disparity.

	MA		TA		
Examples	Cyl (D)	Flat Axis (°)	Cyl (D)	Flat Axis (°)	Classification
1	−1.00	175	1.50	178	Normal
2	−3.50	45	4.00	37	Normal
3	−1.25	80	1.75	60	Abnormal
4	−2.50	005	1.75	170	Abnormal
5	−3.75	130	3.00	125	Normal
6	−1.75	180	0.25	180	Abnormal

(MA: manifest astigmatism; TA: tomographic astigmatism)

There are several factors of astigmatic disparity:

- *Lenticular astigmatism:* It is the most common cause of astigmatic disparity.
- *Cataract:* Early cataract can be missed during the initial exam, hence the importance of a detailed dilated exam.
- Ectatic corneal diseases.
- Irregular corneal or lenticular astigmatism.
- Contact lenses.
- Misalignment.
- *Tear film disturbance:* Especially dry eye.
- Corneal opacities.
- Previous corneal surgeries.
- Bad quality of the capture.
- *Large angle kappa:* A rare cause.

In the case of astigmatic disparity, the decision to treat astigmatism depends on the following nine probabilities:

1. TA and MA are with-the-rule (WTR) and the magnitude of the former is more than the latter.
2. TA and MA are WTR and the magnitude of the former is less than the latter.
3. TA and MA are against-the-rule (ATR) and the magnitude of the former is more than the latter.
4. TA and MA are ATR and the magnitude of the former is less than the latter.
5. TA is WTR and MA is ATR with the magnitude of the former is more than the latter.
6. TA is WTR and MA is ATR with the magnitude of the former is less than the latter.
7. TA is ATR and MA is WTR with the magnitude of the former is more than the latter.
8. TA is ATR and MA is WTR with the magnitude of the former is less than the latter.
9. TA and/or MA are oblique with more than 15° difference between their axes.

NB: The astigmatism is considered as WTR when the *steep* axis is 90°±15°, ATR when the *steep* axis is 180°±15°, and oblique if otherwise.

Table 4.16 summarizes the nine probabilities.

In laser-based refractive surgery, there are general rules that should be followed to avoid or reduce surprises as much as possible. The general rules are:

1. If MA > TA, avoid flipping the WTR TA into ATR TA.
2. If MA > TA, try reducing the difference in magnitude by compensating with the spherical equivalent (SE) without affecting the corrected distance visual acuity (CDVA).
3. If manifest refraction (MR) is modified, plan for enhancement.

Table 4.17 summarizes treatment rules.

Table 4.16: Probabilities of astigmatic disparity.						
				Examples		
Probability	*MA*	*TA*	*Magnitude*	*No.*	*MA*	*TA*
1	WTR	WTR	MA > TA	1	−2.75 × 180	−2.25 × 170
2	WTR	WTR	MA < TA	2	−1.75 × 10	−2.50 × 180
3	ATR	ATR	MA > TA	3A	−2.00 × 80	−1.25 × 95
	ATR	ATR	MA > TA	3B	−2.75 × 80	−1.25 × 95
4	ATR	ATR	MA < TA	4	−2.50 × 100	−3.00 × 95
5	ATR	WTR	MA > TA	5	−1.25 × 85	−0.50 × 165
6	ATR	WTR	MA < TA	6	−1.00 × 80	−1.75 × 180
7	WTR	ATR	MA > TA	7	−1.25 × 175	−0.25 × 90
8	WTR	ATR	MA < TA	8	−0.50 × 180	−0.75 × 85
9	MA, TA or both are oblique		Regardless	9	−0.75 × 55	−1.00 × 95

(ATR: against the rule; WTR: with the rule; MA: manifest astigmatism; TA: tomographic astigmatism)

Table 4.17: Treatment rules in astigmatic disparity.

Probability	Treatment Rules	Example
1	Correct the magnitude of TA on the MA axis and compensate with the SE[a]	1
2	Correct the MA	2
3	MA–TA ≤1 D: correct the MA[a]	3A
	MA–TA >1 D: correct the magnitude of TA on the MA axis + 1 D and compensate for the residual by SE[a]	3B
4	Correct the MA	4
5	Recheck refraction, use the least possible magnitude of MA and compensate by SE[a]	5
6	Recheck refraction, use the least possible magnitude of MA and compensate by SE[a]	6
7	Recheck refraction, use the least possible magnitude of MA and compensate by SE[a]	7
8	Recheck refraction, use the least possible magnitude of MA and compensate by SE[a]	8
9	Correct the MA[a]	9

(MA: manifest astigmatism; SE: spherical equivalent; TA: tomographic astigmatism)
[a]Plan for enhancement

Example 1:
Manifest refraction (MR) = –1.00 D sph/–2.75 D cyl × 180
TA = –2.25 D cyl × 170
Plan: –1.25 D sph/–2.00 D cyl × 180.
NB: The patient may need enhancement.

Example 2:
MR = –0.50 D sph/–1.75 D cyl × 10
TA = –2.50 D cyl × 180
Plan: –0.50 D sph/–1.75 D cyl × 10

Example 3A:
MR = − 0.50 D sph/−2.00 D cyl × 80
TA = − 1.25 D cyl × 95
Plan: − 0.50 D sph/−2.00 D cyl × 80
NB: The patient may need enhancement.

Example 3B:
MR = −0.50 D sph/−2.75 D cyl × 80
TA = −1.25 D cyl × 95
Plan: −0.75 D sph/−2.25 D cyl × 80
NB: The patient may need enhancement.

Example 4:
MR = −1.00 D sph/−2.50 D cyl × 100
TA = −3.00 D cyl × 95
Plan: −1.00 D sph/−2.50 D cyl × 100

Example 5:
MR = +0.75 D sph/−1.25 D cyl × 85
TA = −0.50 D cyl × 165
Plan: Recheck, use the least magnitude of astigmatism, and compensate with the SE; e.g. +0.50 D sph/−0.75 D cyl × 85
NB: The patient may need enhancement.

Example 6:
MR = −1.50 D sph/−1.00 D cyl × 80
TA = −1.75 D cyl × 180
Plan: Recheck, use the least magnitude of astigmatism, and compensate with the SE; e.g. −1.75 D sph/−0.50 D cyl × 80
NB: The patient may need enhancement.

Example 7:
MR = +0.50 D sph/−1.25 D cyl × 170
TA = −0.25 D cyl × 90
Plan: Recheck, use the least magnitude of astigmatism, and compensate with the SE; e.g. +0.25 D sph/−0.75 D cyl × 170
NB: The patient may need enhancement.

Example 8:
MR = –3.00 D sph/–0.50 D cyl × 180
TA = –0.75 D cyl × 85
Plan: Recheck, use the least magnitude of astigmatism, and compensate with the SE; e.g. –3.25 D sph
NB: The patient may need enhancement.

Example 9:
MR = –4.00 D sph/–0.75 D cyl × 55
TA = –1.00 D cyl × 95
Plan: MR = –4.00 D sph/–0.75 D cyl × 55
NB: The patient may need enhancement.

Tomographic Rules in Lens-based Refractive Surgery Options

Lens-based refractive surgery consists of Phakic Intraocular Lens (PIOL) implantation, and Clear Lens Extraction (CLE) or Refractive Lens Exchange (RLE) with Intraocular Lens (IOL) implantation. The IOLs used in the CLE are either Monofocal or Premium lenses, including Multifocal, Trifocal, and Extended Depth of Focus (EDOF) lenses.

Corneal tomography and wavefront should be studied systematically to reveal any corneal irregularity or inter-eye asymmetry. Corneal irregularity should be detected before lens-based refractive surgery because:

- It may result from dry eye disease (DED) and ocular surface disease (OSD), which must be properly and adequately treated before any type of refractive surgery.
- It is the main reason for inaccurate measurements of K-readings and, therefore, IOL calculations. Such inaccurate measurements could have been reduced if the irregularity was diagnosed before that surgery. Reduction of errors can be achieved by treating the reasons of irregularity if possible, such as treating DED and OSD, and by using different methods of measurements. Moreover, a proper consent form can be prepared.
- It leads to bad quality and quantity of postoperative visual acuity. That occurs because of the inaccurate K-readings and IOL calculations, and because of the associated higher-order aberrations (HOAs).
- It may result from ectatic corneal diseases (ECDs).

- It may result from previous corneal refractive surgery. As mentioned in Chapter 3, the most useful maps for detection and differentiation are the anterior tangential map and the relative pachymetry map.
- It induces dysphotopsia, especially after premium IOL implantation. Corneal irregularity is the main reason for postoperative failure and premium IOL extraction.

■ RULES IN PHAKIC IOL IMPLANTATION

There are several factors to be considered in PIOL implantation, including the exclusion of ocular pathologies and systemic contraindications, age, profession, demands, type and magnitude of refractive error, uncorrected and corrected visual acuity, corneal tomography, ocular aberrometry, specular microscopy, and horizontal white-to-white (HWTW) or horizontal sulcus-to-sulcus (HSTS) diameter. Recently, some PIOL formulas depend on scleral spur to scleral spur (SS-SS) diameter. Moreover, the amount of astigmatism determines the type of PIOL (aspheric vs. toric).

Corneal tomography should be studied for the following purposes:

- *To check corneal regularity:* Study the anterior sagittal curvature map and corneal wavefront. When the cornea is irregular (RMS is abnormal), and the patient has symptoms, visual function after PIOL implantation may be suboptimal. The more severe the irregularity, the more defected the desired visual function. However, corneal irregularity is not a contraindication to this type of refractive surgery as toric PIOLs can be implanted in keratoconic and ectatic eyes, but after considering how significant the difference between corrected (CDVA) and uncorrected (UDVA) distance visual acuity. For example, if the preoperative UDVA = 0.1 and CDVA = 0.7, implanting a toric IOL is reasonable. If UDVA = 0.2 and CDVA = 0.4, implanting a toric IOL is irrelevant.

- *To look for two tomographic parameters (**Fig. 5.1** blue ellipses):*
  - *Anterior chamber depth (ACD):* ACD (External) is measured from corneal epithelium (includes central cornea thickness), while ACD (Internal) is measured from corneal endothelium, both to the anterior surface of the crystalline lens. The external ACD is needed for PIOL calculations, while the internal ACD is the indicator of to-do or not-to-do.
  - *Anterior chamber angle (ACA):* For anterior chamber PIOL implantation (e.g., Artisan), the ACD should be ≥3.0 mm, while for the posterior chamber PIOL implantation (e.g., ICL and IPCL), the ACD should be ≥2.8 mm. In both types, the ACA should be ≥30°.
  - *Anterior chamber volume (ACV):* For both types of PIOLs, the ACV should be ≥100 mm³.
- PIOLs are implanted in the sulcus. Therefore, HWTW or HSTS are crucial to achieve a vault (distance between the PIOL and the anterior surface of the crystalline lens) of 300–600 µm. Holladay report in the Pentacam displays HWTW diameter, as shown in **Figure 5.2** (red ellipse). However, HWTW is more accurately measured by optical devices. The normal range of HWTW diameter is 11–13 mm.
- If the corneal thickness spatial profile (CTSP) and percentage thickness increase (PTI) are available and show flat patterns, cornea guttata and Fuchs' dystrophy should be suspected. However, specular microscopy is mandatory before all types of lens-based refractive surgery.

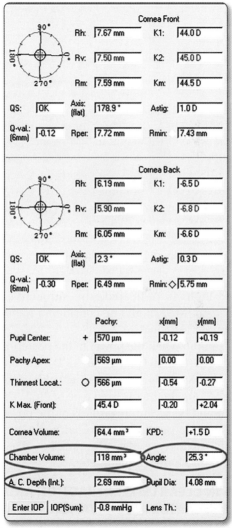

Fig. 5.1: Tomographic parameters for phakic IOL implantation.

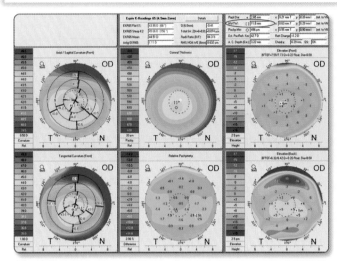

Fig. 5.2: Holladay report. The horizontal white-to-white (HWTW) diameter (red ellipse).

- If toric PIOL is indicated, the subjective manifest astigmatism (MA) should be considered rather than the tomographic astigmatism.
- *Mesopic pupil:* When the power of the posterior chamber type of PIOL is high (more than –5 D), the optic part of the lens is thick. This may cause night glare if the mesopic pupil is >7 mm. In the iris fixed type of PIOL, the mesopic pupil should be <7 mm regardless of the power because large mesopic pupils interfere with the stability and centration of this type. Mesopic pupil should be measured by an infrared-based pupillometer.

RULES IN CLEAR LENS EXTRACTION AND MONOFOCAL IOL IMPLANTATION

Many factors should be taken into consideration when planning for this type of refractive surgery. They include exclusion of ocular pathologies and systemic contra-indications, age, profession, demands, type and magnitude of refractive error, visual acuity, determination of the non-dominant eye, positive tolerance test, corneal tomography, corneal aberrometry, specular microscopy, and HWTW or HSTS diameter.

Corneal tomography and wavefront should be studied for the following purposes:

- To check corneal regularity by studying the anterior sagittal curvature map and corneal wavefront. Study the total RMS of the five main HOAs and the Zernike coefficient (ZC) of the SA **(Fig. 5.3)**. This step is important for selecting the best IOL type and predicting the quality of the postoperative vision.

- To investigate any previous corneal surgery. The anterior tangential curvature map and the relative pachymetry map are used for this purpose. In the case of previous corneal surgeries, simulated keratometric readings (Sim-Ks) are no longer valid. If the previous operation was myopic treatment, Sim-Ks are underestimated, which leads to a hyperopic shift in postoperative outcomes, and vice versa after hyperopic treatment, where Sim-Ks are overestimated. In such cases, the most reliable method for Keratometric reading (K-reading) measurements is the equivalent K-reading (EKR) in the Holladay report. Jack Holladay recommends using K_1 and K_2 in the 4.5-mm zone centered with pupil center, as shown in **Figure 5.4**. Moreover, special formulas are available and recommended to avoid errors in IOL calculation, such as Barret-Universal-2 formula in which the EKR readings are used. However, it is highly recommended to check the IOL power by more than one method and compare the results with the recommendations given by the ASCRS online calculator *http://iolcalc.ascrs.org/wbfrmCalculator.aspx*.

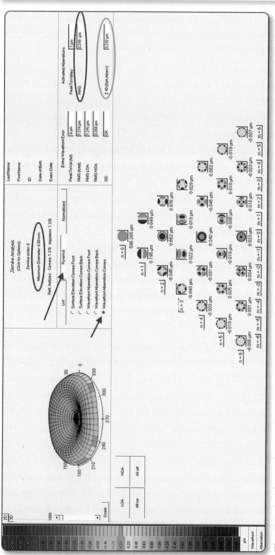

Fig. 5.3: Studying the total RMS of higher-order aberrations (HOAs), consisting of the 3rd order and the spherical aberration (SA). The standard settings are 6 mm of maximum diameter (red ellipse) and wavefront of both surfaces (red arrow). The pyramid display is easier to read (blue arrow). The RMS of the selected HOAs is displayed in the blue ellipse and the individual SA Zernike coefficient is displayed in the green ellipse.

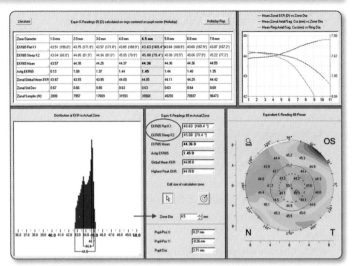

Fig. 5.4: The equivalent K-reading (EKR) (red ellipse) in the Holladay report. The standard zone, as recommended by Jack Holladay, is the 4.5-mm zone (red arrow).

- To check the ACD. The average range of ACD is 2.5–4 mm when measured centrally and internally (endothelium to anterior capsular bag). ACD is usually out of this range in the case of axial ametropia. In other words, when ACD is out of the average range, the axial length is usually out of the normal range as well. Regardless of the axial length, abnormal ACD necessitates the use of special formulas to calculate the IOL because the traditional formulas are calibrated based on an average range of ACD. Modern IOL formulas take into consideration the effective lens position (ELP) related to ACD and crystalline lens thickness.
- To select the best IOL type. Follow the Practical Subjective IOL Selection (PSIS) algorithm (Chapter 2).

- *The posterior corneal astigmatism:* It should be considered in Toric IOL calculation because it affects the calculations if >0.50 D. In the conventional IOL calculation formulas, posterior corneal astigmatism is not considered. Such formulas assume that the keratometric method for K-reading measurements compensates for the effect of posterior corneal power by using the keratometric index (1.3375) instead of the true refractive index of corneal stroma (1.376). Such an assumption is not always accurate. In toric IOL measurements, if the posterior corneal astigmatism is not taken into account, overcorrection results in the case of with-the-rule (WTR) anterior corneal astigmatism and undercorrection results in the case of against-the-rule (ATR) anterior corneal astigmatism. Moreover, there is a proportional relationship between posterior astigmatism and WTR anterior astigmatism, while there is no relationship in the case of ATR anterior astigmatism. In other words, the higher the magnitude of WTR anterior astigmatism, the higher the magnitude of posterior astigmatism, while the magnitude of posterior astigmatism is not affected by the magnitude of the anterior ATR astigmatism. Those factors make it necessary to involve posterior astigmatism into the measurements. That can be achieved by using modern formulas that depend on the true corneal astigmatism measured by the total corneal refractive power (TCRP). The TCRP takes into account anterior and posterior corneal surfaces, corneal thickness, and the true refractive corneal index, and uses Snell's law (ray tracing). **Figure 5.5** represents the power distribution, including the TCRP (red ellipse). The values should be studied in "ring" rather than "zone" and centered with the "apex" rather than the "pupil" (blue arrows). The K-readings of the

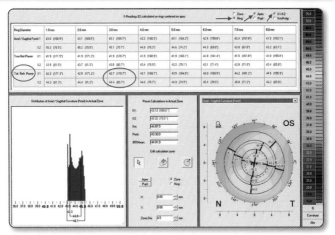

Fig. 5.5: The total corneal refractive power (TCRP) (red ellipse). The true K-readings display (red arrow). The settings are ring/apex (blue arrows) at 3 mm (blue ellipse).

3-mm ring are considered for IOL calculations (blue ellipse). Those K-readings should not be used in the traditional formulas as there are special formulas for toric IOLs.

- True corneal astigmatism. It is studied by the TCRP in the 3-mm ring centered on apex, as shown in **Figure 5.6**. It is essential to check any astigmatic disparity and to decide incision type, shape, size, and location after considering the surgically-induced astigmatism (SIA), which is subjective to each surgeon. The induction of SIA is subject to the following rules:
  - The farther the incision from the visual axis, the less the flattening effect.
  - The more symmetric the incision, the less the flattening effect.
  - Scleral incisions have a less flattening effect than limbal and clear corneal incisions.

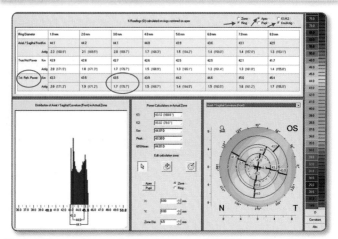

Fig. 5.6: The total corneal refractive power (TCRP) (red ellipse). The true corneal astigmatism display (red arrow). The settings are ring/apex (blue arrows) at 3 mm (blue ellipse).

- Scleral bent frown incision has a less flattening effect than the arcuate scleral incision.
- Limbal (vascular, near-clear corneal) incisions have a less flattening effect than avascular, truly clear corneal incisions.
- Temporal incisions and oblique-meridian incisions have a less flattening effect than superior incisions because they have less influence from the eyelid and extraocular muscle and are farther from the center of the cornea. In elderly patients with ATR astigmatism, the flattening effect of the temporal incision is an advantage.
- Oblique-meridian incisions have a less flattening effect than superior incisions.
- The narrower and the longer the tunnel of incision, the less flattening effect it induces.

- Arcuate corneal incisions have a more flattening effect than straight linear corneal incisions. If arcuate incisions are performed on the steep axis in the case of small preoperative astigmatism, astigmatism will be overcorrected.

- Although the IOL is implanted in the bag in this type of refractive surgery, HWTW or HSTS is crucial to determine the haptic diameter of the IOL. The average HWTW diameter is 11–13 mm. In extreme refractive errors, the ocular axial length is usually abnormal, and the anatomical features of the anterior segment are also abnormal. When the eye is long, HWTW is larger than average and vice versa when the eye is short. Conventional IOLs have specific haptic-to-haptic diameters. Implantation of IOLs with the conventional diameters may lead to IOL decentration when the eye is long (large capsular diameter), or to glaucoma when the eye is short (small capsular diameter) because of the forward bending of the IOL, leading to pupillary block. Therefore, when the HWTW is out of average, the haptic-to-haptic diameter should be customized. Holladay report in the Pentacam displays HWTW diameter, as shown in **Figure 5.2**. However, HWTW is more accurately measured by optical devices.

- If the corneal thickness spatial profile (CTSP) and percentage thickness increase (PTI) are available and show flat patterns, cornea guttata and Fuchs' dystrophy should be suspected. However, specular microscopy is mandatory before all types of lens-based refractive surgery.

- Consider the TCRP astigmatism rather than the MA because the lenticular component is removed in this type of refractive surgery.

RULES IN CLEAR LENS EXTRACTION AND PREMIUM LENS IMPLANTATION

Factors affecting the decision in this type of refractive surgery are ocular pathologies and systemic contraindications, age, profession, demands, type and magnitude of refractive error, visual acuity, determination of the non-dominant eye, corneal tomography, corneal aberrometry, specular microscopy, and HWTW or HSTS diameter.

Corneal tomography should be studied for the following purposes:

- To check corneal regularity by studying the anterior sagittal curvature map and corneal wavefront. Study the total RMS of the five main HOAs. If the total RMS is >0.35 μm, premium lenses are contraindicated unless the HOAs are treated by customized laser vision correction, and the RMS became normal before implanting the premium IOLs. However, if dysphotopsia develops after premium IOL implantation due to missed preoperative HOAs, customized laser vision correction can be applied before deciding to explant the premium IOL.

- To investigate any previous corneal surgery, as mentioned above.

- *True corneal astigmatism:* This is essential in this type of refractive surgery for two reasons:
  1. If the TCRP astigmatism is >0.50, the efficacy of the premium IOL, and therefore the quality of vision, will be affected. The patient may experience dysphotopsia postoperatively unless a toric premium IOL is implanted or the astigmatism is treated.
  2. To decide the incision type, shape, size, and location after considering the SIA, as mentioned above.

- Measurement of HWTW or HSTS is important in this type of refractive surgery for the same reasons that were mentioned in the previous type. Remember that HWTW is more accurately measured by optical devices.

- *Mesopic pupil:* If the mesopic pupil is <2 mm or >6 mm, premium lenses are contraindicated. The mesopic pupil should be measured by an infrared-based pupillometer.

- *Angle kappa:* A Premium IOL perfectly functions when it is centered on the visual axis. The IOL is usually implanted in the capsular bag; therefore, the center of the IOL will automatically centralize on the geometric center of the capsule, which is approximately correspondent to the pupil center rather than the visual axis. When angle kappa is very small, the visual axis is very close to the pupil center, and the premium IOL functions ideally. The larger the angle, the less the efficacy of the IOL. When angle kappa is within the normal range (≤ 200 µm), the difference between the geometrical center of the capsular bag and the visual axis is insignificant, and the quality of vision is optimum. When the angle is 200–400 µm, the difference may cause mild dysphotopsia which is usually compensated by neural adaptation within six months. When the angle is >400 µm, premium IOL implantation is contraindicated because the difference is significant, and dysphotopsia will be intolerable. Dysphotopsia is the primary reason for premium IOL explantation.

- If the corneal thickness spatial profile (CTSP) and percentage thickness increase (PTI) are available and show flat patterns, cornea guttata and Fuchs' dystrophy should be suspected. However, specular microscopy is mandatory before all types of lens-based refractive surgery.

- Consider the TCRP astigmatism rather than the MA because the lenticular component is removed in this type of refractive surgery.

Corneal Tomography in Cataract Surgery

Corneal tomography is an essential screening tool before modern cataract surgery. A successful cataract surgery depends not only on accurate measurements of the axial length, but on many other factors such as corneal surface; corneal regularity; anterior and posterior corneal astigmatism; previous corneal surgery; pupil size; angle kappa; horizontal white-to-white (HWTW) diameter; anterior chamber depth (ACD); incision type, shape, size, and location; and corneal wavefront. Such factors should be appropriately studied to make an accurate cataract plan. In general, the workup for cataract surgery is very similar to the workup for clear lens extraction that was discussed in detail in Chapter 5, with some differences to be highlighted in this chapter.

■ DETECTING CORNEAL IRREGULARITY

Corneal tomography should be studied systematically, similar to refractive surgery, to reveal any corneal irregularity or inter-eye asymmetry. Corneal irregularity should be detected before cataract surgery because:

- It may result from dry eye disease (DED) and ocular surface disease (OSD), which must be properly and adequately treated before cataract surgery.
- It is the main reason for inaccurate measurements of K-readings and, therefore, intraocular lens (IOL) calculations. Such inaccurate measurements could have been reduced if the irregularity was diagnosed

before that surgery. Reduction of errors can be achieved by treating the reasons of irregularity if possible, such as DED and OSD, and by using different methods of measurements. Moreover, a proper consent form can be prepared.

- It leads to bad quality and quantity of postoperative visual acuity. That occurs because of the inaccurate K-readings and IOL calculations, and because of the associated higher-order aberrations (HOAs).

- It may result from ectatic corneal diseases (ECDs). In the case of an ECD, the plan of cataract surgery may differ whether the cataract procedure is to be performed first or the ECD is to be managed first. In addition, special formulas for IOL calculation should be used. The diagnosis of ECDs before cataract surgery makes the plan clear and can be discussed properly with the patient, and a proper consent form can be prepared.

- It induces dysphotopsia, especially after premium IOL implantation. Corneal irregularity is the main reason for postoperative failure and premium IOL explantation. However, if dysphotopsia develops after premium IOL implantation due to missed preoperative HOAs, customized laser vision correction can be applied before deciding to explant the premium IOL.

Corneal irregularity is evaluated by studying the anterior sagittal curvature map and corneal wavefront. Corneal irregularity is considered significant if the total RMS of HOAs is >0.35 μm.

■ MEASURING TRUE CORNEAL ASTIGMATISM

It is essential for premium IOL implantation. As mentioned in Chapter 5, if the TCRP astigmatism is >0.50, the efficacy of the premium IOL, and therefore the quality of vision, will be affected, and the patient may experience dysphotopsia postoperatively unless a toric premium IOL is implanted or the astigmatism is treated.

MEASURING POSTERIOR CORNEAL ASTIGMATISM

It is essential for toric IOL implantation, as mentioned in Chapter 5.

DETECTING PREVIOUS CORNEAL SURGERIES

Previous corneal surgeries should be detected by using the anterior tangential map and the relative pachymetry map. In the case of previous corneal surgeries, the most reliable method for K-reading measurements in such cases is the equivalent K-reading (EKR) in the Holladay report. Jack Holladay recommends using K_1 and K_2 in the 4.5-mm zone centered with pupil center, as mentioned in Chapter 5. Moreover, special formulas are available and recommended in such cases to avoid errors in IOL calculation, such as Barret-Universal-2 formula in which the EKR readings are used. However, it is highly recommended to check the IOL power by more than one method and compare the results with the recommendations given by the ASCRS online calculator *http://iolcalc.ascrs.org/wbfrmCalculator.aspx*.

PUPIL SIZE

If the mesopic pupil is <2 mm or >6 mm, premium lenses are contraindicated. The mesopic pupil should be measured by an infrared-based pupillometer.

■ ANGLE KAPPA

As mentioned in Chapter 5, premium IOL implantation is contraindicated when angle kappa is >400 μm because of the risk of intolerable-induced dysphotopsia.

■ HORIZONTAL WHITE-TO-WHITE DIAMETER (HWTW)

Measuring the HWTW diameter is essential, especially in abnormal axial lengths, as mentioned in Chapter 5.

■ ANTERIOR CHAMBER DEPTH (ACD)

Anterior chamber depth should be considered when measuring the IOL, especially when the ACD is abnormal, as mentioned in Chapter 5.

■ INCISION TYPE, SHAPE, SIZE AND LOCATION

This was discussed in Chapter 5.

■ IOL TYPE

Selecting the best type of IOL depends on three factors:
1. Patient's demands (depth of focus vs. quality of the image).
2. The RMS of HOAs.
3. The Zernike coefficient (ZC) of the spherical aberration (SA).

Follow the PSIS algorithm (Chapter 2; **Figs. 2.44 to 2.47**).

■ TREATMENT OF ASTIGMATISM

Consider the TCRP astigmatism rather than the manifest astigmatism (MA) becasue the lenticular component is removed in cataract surgery.

ASTIGMATIC KERATOTOMY (AK) AND LIMBAL RELAXING INCISIONS (LRIs)

Such procedures are sometimes planned with the cataract procedure. Corneal tomography is essential before such procedures:

- To guide the number, length, depth, and location of the incisions. They are determined by the magnitude and type of astigmatism (WTR, ATR, or oblique) in addition to the patient's age.

- In astigmatism with skewed radial axis (SRAX), the cornea does not normally respond to AK and LRIs, and they may induce more irregularity.

- To customize the incisions. It is not uncommon to encounter an asymmetric bowtie (AB) that cannot be recognized by the keratometer. In the AB pattern, the incision on the steeper side can be made a little longer than on the other side. In symmetric bowtie with SRAX (SB/SRAX) and AB/SRAX patterns, incisions should not be done on opposite sides but should be placed at the tips of astigmatism to round it out and make it more symmetrical. That can be planned by tomography and topography rather than keratometry.

- Tomography can give regional pachymetry values in the areas where the relaxing incisions are planned; therefore, the depth of incisions can precisely be calculated.

- Prohibiting AK and LRIs when the sagittal curvature map shows an unspecific irregular pattern.

Special nomograms are available to guide this procedure, such as the NAPA nomogram.

■ CORNEA GUTTATA AND FUCHS' DYSTROPHY

If the corneal thickness spatial profile (CTSP) and percentage thickness increase (PTI) are available and show flat patterns, cornea guttata and Fuchs' dystrophy should be suspected. However, specular microscopy is highly recommended as a part of the preoperative workup in all cases of cataract.

CORNEAL TOMOGRAPHY AND WAVEFRONT FOR FOLLOW-UP

They should be performed after cataract surgery when the postoperative corrected distance visual acuity (CDVA) is not optimal for no apparent reason. Corneal irregularities and HOAs are the first to be suspected. Moreover, if the incision was sutured, removal of the sutures can be guided by tomography.

Tomography-based Decision Making in Cataract and Refractive Surgery

This chapter is a review of the steps to follow in the workup for refractive surgery and cataract surgery based on tomographic data. Readers are recommended to consider this chapter as a checklist.

DECISION MAKING IN LASER-BASED REFRACTIVE SURGERY

Step 1: Study Tomography Systematically

- Validate the maps.
  - Check quality specification (Qs).
  - Check misalignment.
  - Check astigmatic disparity.
- Exclude factors of false positives and false negatives.
- Apply the practical subjective scoring system (PS3).
- Study the relative pachymetry map to rule out any previous corneal refractive surgery.
- Study pachymetric profiles to inspect for cornea guttata and Fuchs dystrophy.
- Study corneal wavefront if the patient has symptoms, the corrected visual acuity is not optimum, or there are some tomographic irregularities. Consider customized laser vision correction in the case of *abnormal symptomatic* higher-order aberrations.

Step 2: Consider Refractive Error Magnitude

- Check if the magnitude is within the recommended range of correction.

- Check if the mesopic pupil diameter is <7 mm.
- Calculate spherical equivalent (SE) and total refraction (TR).
- Consider cyclotorsion compensation when the astigmatic correction is ≥1.50 D.
- Consider the recentration technique, when angle kappa is > 200 μm.

Step 3: Make the Calculations for Thickness and K-readings

- *For surface ablation:*
  - Consider the preoperative central corneal thickness (CCT). Be committed to the limits.
  - Use TR for thickness calculations.
  - Decide the optical zone (OZ). Consider the mesopic pupil diameter.
  - Calculate the central ablation depth (CAD).
  - Calculate the postoperative CCT. Be committed to the limits.
  - Use SE for K-reading calculations.
  - Calculate the postoperative anterior mean K (Km). Be committed to the limits.
- *For LASIK and FemtoLASIK:*
  - Consider the preoperative CCT. Be committed to the limits.
  - Use TR for thickness calculations.
  - Decide the OZ. Consider the mesopic pupil diameter.
  - Calculate the CAD.
  - Calculate percent tissue altered (PTA). Be committed to the limits.
  - Use SE for K-reading calculations.
  - Calculate the postoperative Km. Be committed to the limits.

- *For SMILE:*
  - Consider the preoperative CCT. Be committed to the limits.
  - Decide OZ, cap thickness, side cut, and bed thickness.
  - Calculate the postoperative CCT. Be committed to the limits.
  - Use SE for K-reading calculations.
  - Calculate the postoperative Km. Be committed to the limits.

Step 4: Perform the Astigmatic Study

- Calculate tomographic astigmatism (TA). Consider the true corneal astigmatism taken from the total corneal refractive power (TCRP) at 3 mm ring/apex. If the TCRP is not available, calculate the magnitude of TA by subtracting the posterior *absolute* value from the anterior *absolute* value and use the flat axis of the later.
- Compare the TCRP astigmatism with the subjective manifest astigmatism (MA).
- In case of disparity, investigate the reasons and follow the rules of the nine probabilities.

Step 5: Study Both Eyes

- Perform the inter-eye asymmetry scoring.
- Check for Forme Fruste Keratoconus (FFKC) and Keratoconus Suspect (KCS).
- Accept the abnormal skewed radial axis index (SRAX) in the case of large angle kappa (> 200 μm) or enantiomorphism.
- In the case of mono-ocular corneal irregularities, exclude corneal pathologies, such as scars and dystrophies.

DECISION MAKING IN LENS-BASED REFRACTIVE SURGERY

Step 1: Study Tomography

- Validate the maps.
- Exclude factors of false positives and false negatives.
- Study tomography systematically, check regularity, and rule out ectatic corneal diseases (ECDs).
- Study the relative pachymetry map to rule out any previous corneal refractive surgery.
- Study pachymetric profiles to inspect for cornea guttata and Fuchs dystrophy.

Step 2: Study Parameters

- *For Phakic IOL (PIOL) implantation:*
  - Study the internal anterior chamber depth, anterior chamber angle, and anterior chamber volume.
  - Measure the horizontal white-to-white (HWTW) diameter.
  - Consider the mesopic pupil diameter.
  - Consider MA rather than tomographic astigmatism.
- *For clear lens extraction (CLE):*
  - Consider the mesopic pupil diameter for Premium IOL implantation.
  - Pay attention to abnormal ACD for IOL calculations.
  - Pay attention to posterior corneal astigmatism for Toric IOL and Premium IOL calculations.
  - Pay attention to the TCRP true corneal astigmatism for Toric IOL and Premium IOL implantation. Consider the surgically induced astigmatism (SIA) and incision type, shape, size, and location.

- Measure the HWTW diameter.
- Consider angle kappa for Premium IOL implantation.
- Consider TCRP astgmatism rather than MA.

Step 3: Study Corneal Wavefront

- In PIOL implantation, study the total RMS, which includes the 3rd order (horizontal and vertical coma, horizontal and vertical trefoil), and the spherical aberration (SA).
- In Monofocal IOL implantation, study the total RMS and the ZC of the SA. Consider patient's demands (depth of focus vs. vision quality). Follow the PSIS algorithm for the best suitable IOL type.
- In Premium IOL implantation, study the total RMS. Consider patient's demands (depth of focus vs. vision quality). Follow the PSIS algorithm.

Step 4: Study Both Eyes

- Check for FFKC and KCS.
- In the case of mono-ocular corneal irregularities, exclude corneal pathologies, such as scars and dystrophies.
- In some cases, lens-based refractive surgery may be suitable for one eye but not for the other eye, or a type is suitable for one eye while another type is suitable for the other eye. In such cases, the plan for both eyes must be clear and discussed with the patient.

■ DECISION MAKING IN CATARACT SURGERY

Step 1: Study Tomography

- Validate the maps.
- Exclude factors of false positives and false negatives.

- Study tomography systematically, check regularity, and rule out ECDs.
- Study the relative pachymetry map to rule out any previous corneal refractive surgery.
- Study pachymetric profiles to inspect for cornea guttata and Fuchs dystrophy.

Step 2: Study Parameters

- Consider the mesopic pupil diameter for Premium IOL implantation.
- Pay attention to abnormal ACD for IOL calculations.
- Pay attention to posterior corneal astigmatism for Toric IOL and Premium IOL calculations.
- Pay attention to the TCRP true corneal astigmatism for Toric IOL and Premium IOL implantation. Consider the SIA and incision type, shape, size, and location.
- Pay attention to the TCRP true corneal astigmatism if astigmatic keratotomy (AK) or limbal-relaxing incisions (LRIs) are planned.
- Measure the HWTW diameter.
- Consider angle kappa for Premium IOL implantation.
- Consider TCRP astigmatism rather than MA.

Step 3: Study Corneal Wavefront

- In Monofocal IOL implantation, study the total RMS and the ZC of the SA. Consider patient's demands (depth of focus vs. vision quality). Follow the PSIS algorithm for the best suitable IOL type.
- In Premium IOL implantation, study the total RMS. Consider patient's demands (depth of focus vs. vision quality). Follow the PSIS algorithm.

Step 4: Study Both Eyes

- Check for FFKC and KCS.
- In the case of mono-ocular corneal irregularities, exclude corneal pathologies, such as scars and dystrophies.
- In some cases, some IOL types may be suitable for one eye but not for the other eye. In such cases, a clear plan for both eyes must be made and discussed with the patient.
- In the case of a unilateral cataract, a plan for both eyes must be clear and discussed with the patient.

Clinical Cases

■ CASE 1

A 35-year-old male visiting for refractive surgery. His subjective refraction is shown in **Table 8.1.1**, and his 4-composite refractive maps are shown in **Figures 8.1.1 and 8.1.2**.

Table 8.1.1: Subjective refraction.				
	Sph (D)	**Cyl (D)**	**Axis**	**CDVA**
OD	−4.00	−2.00	180°	1.0
OS	−5.00	−1.00	175°	1.0

(CDVA: corrected distance visual acuity measured in decimal)

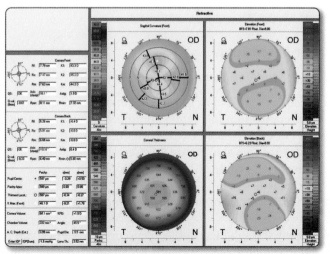

Fig. 8.1.1: The 4-composite map of the right eye.

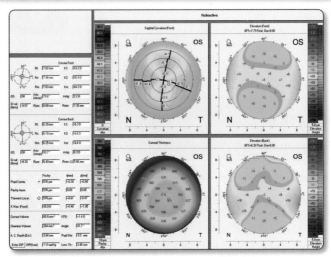

Fig. 8.1.2: The 4-composite map of the left eye.

The patient has no other symptoms, such as glare, halos, ghost images, shadows, or starbursts.

Laser-based Study

Step 1: Studying Tomographic Risk Factors

1. *Validate the maps:* Qs is OK, there is no significant difference in pupil center coordinates between the two eyes ($X + X = -0.29 + 0.30 = +0.01$, $Y - Y = 0.50 - 0.56 = -0.06$) as shown in **Figure 8.1.3**, and there is no astigmatic disparity **(Table 8.1.2)**. Therefore, the captures are accepted.

2. *Exclude factors of false positives and false negatives:* No factors exist.

3. Apply the practical subjective scoring system (PS3) on the available data. **Table 8.1.3** summarizes the study.

	Pachy:	x[mm]	y[mm]		Pachy:	x[mm]	y[mm]
Pupil Center:	+ 597 µm	-0.29	+0.50	Pupil Center:	+ 576 µm	+0.30	+0.56
Pachy Apex:	● 589 µm	0.00	0.00	Pachy Apex:	● 576 µm	0.00	0.00
Thinnest Locat.:	○ 587 µm	-0.34	-0.27	Thinnest Locat.:	○ 570 µm	+0.61	-0.47
K Max. (Front):	◆ 46.1 D	-0.21	+1.78	K Max. (Front):	◆ 45.9 D	+0.40	+1.95

Fig. 8.1.3: Validating the maps by the pupil center coordinates.

Table 8.1.2: Astigmatic disparity.

	MA[a]	TA[a]	Disparity
OD	2.00 × 180°	1.50 × 009°	NO
OS	1.00 × 175°	1.90 × 170°	NO

(MA: manifest astigmatism; TA: tomographical astigmatism)
[a]Astigmatism is displayed in absolute value at the flat axis

Table 8.1.3: The practical subjective scoring system (PS3).

Parameters	OD	OS	Moderate	High
Ant. Km (D)	44.2	44.2	48–50	>50
TCT (µm)	587	570	470–500	<470
Inferior superior asymmetry (D)	S–I = 2.2	S–I = 1.8	I–S ≥1.5 S–I ≥2.5	NA
SRAX	0°	0°	NA	≥22°
Ant. Elevation (µm) @ TL	+6	+2	NA	≥8 emmetropia and myopia; ≥7 hyperopia and mixed astigmatism
Post. Elevation (µm) @ TL	+6	+2	NA	≥18 emmetropia and myopia; ≥28 hyperopia and mixed astigmatism
Pachymetry pattern	Concentric	Concentric	Dome, Droplet	Bell, Globus
Inter-eye asymmetry	Score 3[a]		Score 4	Score 5

(Ant. Km: Mean K on the anterior corneal surface; TCT: thinnest corneal thickness; SRAX: skewed radial axis index; TL: thinnest location; NA: not available; SE: spherical aberration)
[a]See table 8.1.4

Table 8.1.4: Inter-eye asymmetry scoring.

Parameters	OD	OS	*Score*	*Abnormal*
Ant. Km (D)	44.2	44.2	0	≥0.3
Post. Km (D)	−6.6	−6.4	1	≥0.1
TCT (μm)	587	570	1	≥12
Ant. Elevation (μm) @ TL	+6	+2	1	≥2
Post. Elevation (μm) @ TL	+6	+2	0	≥5
Total			3	5

(Ant. Km: mean K on the anterior corneal surface; Post. Km: mean K on posterior corneal surface; TCT: thinnest corneal thickness; TL: thinnest location)

Abnormal values are coded in orange for moderate-risk and red for high-risk factors. The table shows neither moderate-risk nor high-risk factors. **Table 8.1.4** represents the inter-eye asymmetry scoring.

4. Study the relative pachymetry map to rule out any previous corneal refractive surgery. The map is not available in this case.
5. Study pachymetric profiles to inspect for cornea guttata and Fuchs' dystrophy. The profiles are not available in this case.
6. The patient has no symptoms, the corrected distance visual acuity (CDVA) = 1.0, and there is no irregularity on tomography. No need to study corneal wavefront in this regard.

Step 2: Considering Refractive Error Magnitude

1. The refractive error magnitude is within the range of correction for the three types of laser-based procedures.
2. The mesopic pupil is <7 mm in diameter.

Table 8.1.5: Spherical equivalent (SE) and total refraction (TR).

	Sph (D)	Cyl (D)	SE (D)	TR (D)
OD	−4.00	−2.00	−5.00	−6.00
OS	−5.00	−1.00	−5.50	−6.00

(SE: spherical equivalent; TR: total refraction)

3. **Table 8.1.5** shows the spherical equivalent (SE) and the total refraction (TR) for this case.
4. Since the magnitude of the planned astigmatic correction is ≥1.50 D in the right eye, cyclotorsion compensation is recommended.
5. Recentration technique is recommended for two reasons—the astigmatism in OD is ≥1.50 D, and the Y coordinate of angle Kappa is >200 μm in both eyes; (−145 μm, +250 μm) in OD and (+150 μm, +280 μm) in OS. Holladay report is not available in this case; therefore, angle Kappa coordinates are calculated by dividing pupil center coordinates by 2 (*see* **Fig. 8.1.3**).

Step 3: Calculations for Thickness and K-readings

In this case, thickness calculations are done based on:
1. 6.5 mm optical zone (OZ) for all options.
2. 130 μm flap for LASIK and FemtoLASIK.
3. 135 μm cap and 15 μm side cut for SMILE.

   Tables 8.1.6 to 8.1.8 show calculations for PRK/surface ablation, LASIK/FemtoLASIK, and SMILE, respectively.

   Table 8.1.9 represents K-reading calculations for laser-based procedures.

Step 4: Astigmatic Study

The total corneal refractive power (TCRP) is not available in this case. Therefore, the tomographic astigmatism (TA) is

Table 8.1.6: Thickness calculations for PRK/surface ablation.

	TR (D)	CAD (µm)	Pre-op CCT (µm)	Post-op CCT (µm)	PRK/ Surface Ablation
OD	−6.00	90	589	499	✓
OS	−6.00	90	576	486	✓

(TR: total refraction; CAD: central ablation depth; CCT: central corneal thickness)

Table 8.1.7: Thickness calculations for LASIK/FemtoLASIK.

	TR (D)	CAD (µm)	Pre-op CCT (µm)	PTA	LASIK
OD	−6.00	90	589	37.35%	✓
OS	−6.00	90	576	38.19%	✓

(TR: total refraction; CAD: central ablation depth; CCT: central corneal thickness; PTA: percent tissue altered)

Table 8.1.8: Thickness calculations for SMILE.

	TR (D)	Pre-op CCT (µm)	Lenticule (µm)	Bed (µm)	Post-op CCT (µm)	SMILE
OD	−6.00	589	108	346	481	✓
OS	−6.00	576	108	333	468	✓

(TR: total refraction; CCT: central corneal thickness)

Table 8.1.9: K-reading calculations.

	SE (D)	Pre-op ant. Km (D)	Change (D)	Post-op ant. Km (D)	Laser-based
OD	−5.00	44.2	−4	40.2	✓
OS	−6.00	44.2	−4.4	39.8	✓

(SE: spherical equivalent; ant. Km: mean K on the anterior corneal surface)

considered. There is no astigmatic disparity in both eyes, as shown in **Table 8.1.2**. Probability No. 1 applies for OD, and probability No. 2 applies for OS (see probabilities in Chapter 4).

Step 5: Studying Both Eyes

Studying both eyes shows no inter-eye asymmetry (*see* **Table 8.1.4**), no ectatic corneal diseases (ECDs), and no suspect of corneal pathologies.

Lens-based Study

Step 1: Study Tomography

In the laser-based study, tomography maps were validated, factors of false findings were excluded, ECDs were ruled out. Unfortunately, the relative pachymetry map and the pachymetry profiles are not available in this case.

Step 2: Study Parameters

1. *In Phakic IOL (PIOL) Implantation:*
   - *Anterior chamber (AC) parameters:* As shown in **Figure 8.1.4**, anterior chamber depth (ACD) is measured externally (including corneal thickness) rather than internally. Therefore, the internal ACD is 3.99 – 0.58 (central corneal thickness) = 3.41 mm in OD and 3.94 – 0.57 = 3.37 mm in OS. The anterior chamber angle (ACA) is 45.5° in OD and 41.7° in OS. The anterior chamber volume (ACV) is 222 mm^3 in OD and 204 mm^3 in OS. All values are suitable for both types of PIOL implantation.
   - *Horizontal white-to-white (HWTW) diameter:* Holladay report is not available in this case. However, HWTW is more accurately measured by optical devices.

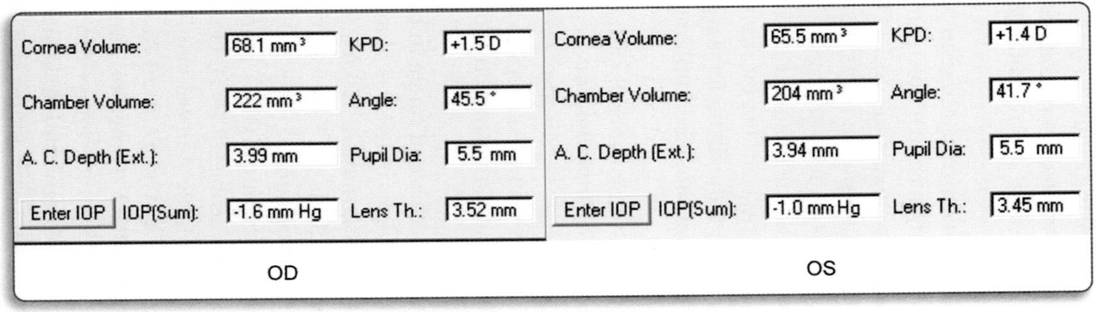

	OD		
Cornea Volume:	68.1 mm³	KPD:	+1.5 D
Chamber Volume:	222 mm³	Angle:	45.5 °
A. C. Depth (Ext.):	3.99 mm	Pupil Dia:	5.5 mm
Enter IOP IOP(Sum):	-1.6 mm Hg	Lens Th.:	3.52 mm

	OS		
Cornea Volume:	65.5 mm³	KPD:	+1.4 D
Chamber Volume:	204 mm³	Angle:	41.7 °
A. C. Depth (Ext.):	3.94 mm	Pupil Dia:	5.5 mm
Enter IOP IOP(Sum):	-1.0 mm Hg	Lens Th.:	3.45 mm

Fig. 8.1.4: Anterior chamber parameters.

- The mesopic pupil is <7 mm.
- Consider MA rather than tomographic astigmatism.

2. *Clear Lens Extraction (CLE) and Monofocal IOL Implantation:*
   - ACD is within the normal range in both eyes, so no special considerations in IOL calculations.
   - The posterior astigmatism is <0.5 D in both eyes, as shown in the 4-composite maps. However, the true corneal astigmatism measured by the TCRP should be considered for IOL calculation. Consider the SIA and incision type, shape, size, and location.
   - *HWTW diameter:* If the diameter is within the normal range, the IOL can safely be implanted; otherwise, a customized haptic-to-haptic diameter is needed.
   - Consider TCRP astigmatism rather than MA.

3. *CLE and Premium IOL Implantation:*
   - Mesopic pupil size is 5.5 mm in both eyes (*see* **Fig. 8.1.4**). It is within the accepted range. However, it is more accurately measured by an infrared-based pupillometer.
   - ACD is within the normal range in both eyes, so no special considerations in IOL calculations.
   - The posterior astigmatism is <0.5 D in both eyes. However, the TCRP is mandatory in the formulas of premium IOL calculation.
   - If a non-toric premium IOL is planned, the TCRP astigmatism should be <0.75 D. Unfortunately, the TCRP is not available, but we can have an idea by calculating the TA. The TA is >0.75 in both eyes, as shown in **Table 8.1.2**. Therefore, non-toric premium IOL is contraindicated unless the astigmatism is treated or a toric-premium IOL is planned. Consider the SIA and incision type, shape, size, and location.

- *HWTW diameter:* If the diameter is within the normal range, the IOL can safely be implanted; otherwise, a customized haptic-to-haptic diameter is needed.
- *Angle kappa:* Based on pupil center coordinates, angle kappa is around (–145 µm, +250 µm) in OD and (+150 µm, +280 µm) in OS. It is within the accepted range.
- Consider TCRP astigmatism rather than MA.

Step 3: Study Corneal Wavefront

1. *In PIOL Implantation:* Although the anterior sagittal curvature map is at low risk (no significant superior, inferior difference and no significant SRAX), corneal wavefront shows high HOAs RMS, mainly on account of the vertical coma. **Figures 8.1.5 and 8.1.6** represent

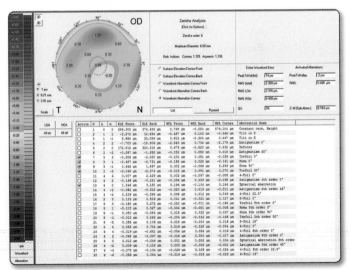

Fig. 8.1.5: Corneal wavefront of the right eye.

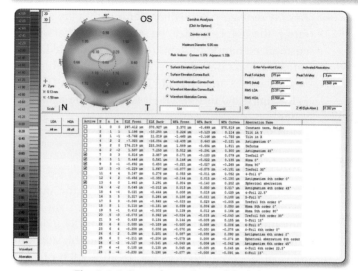

Fig. 8.1.6: Corneal wavefront of the left eye.

corneal wavefront for OD and OS, respectively. Despite this high HOAs RMS, the patient is asymptomatic, which means either neural adaptation to these native HOAs or lenticular compensation. Because in PIOL implantation, the crystalline lens remains intact, those HOAs are not affected, and good results are expected.

2. *CLE and Monofocal IOL Implantation:* The total RMS is >0.35 μm on account of the vertical coma in OD and vertical coma and SA in OS. Following PSIS algorithm **(Fig. 2.44)**, an aspherical IOL with zero-SA is recommended.

3. *CLE and Premium IOL Implantation:* Since the total RMS is >0.35 μm, this type of refractive surgery is contraindicated.

Table 8.1.10: Recommendations in laser-based refractive surgery.

	PRK	LASIK[a]	SMILE[b]	OZ (mm)	Cyclotorsion compensation	Recentration
OD	✓	✓	✓	6.5	✓	✓
OS	✓	✓	✓	6.5	Not necessary	✓

(OZ: optical zone)
[a]Flap ≤ 130 µm
[b]Cap = 135 µm and side cut = 15 µm

Step 4: Study Both Eyes

1. No ECDs in both eyes.
2. No suspect of corneal pathologies.
3. Both eyes are similar in terms of the decision for lens-based refractive surgery. However, it is fundamental to discuss with the patient the expected postoperative quality of vision and DOF in each eye.

Case 1 Summary

Based on Corneal Tomography:

- All types of laser-based refractive surgery are suitable. **Table 8.1.10** represents the recommendations.
- PIOL implantation is suitable with no special precautions.
- CLE and monofocal IOL implantation is suitable, but the quality of postoperative vision will most probably not be optimum.
- CLE and premium IOL implantation is contraindicated.

■ CASE 2

A 27-year-old female visiting for refractive surgery. Her subjective refraction is shown in **Table 8.2.1**, and her 4-composite refractive maps are shown in **Figures 8.2.1 and 8.2.2**.

Table 8.2.1: Subjective refraction.

	Sph (D)	Cyl (D)	Axis	CDVA
OD	−2.50	−3.75	180°	1.0
OS	−3.00	−3.50	180°	1.0

(CDVA: corrected distance visual acuity measured in decimal)

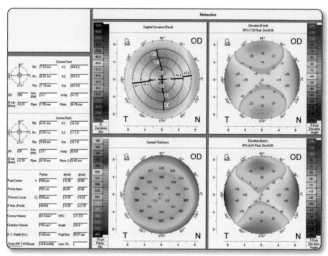

Fig. 8.2.1: The 4-composite map of the right eye.

The patient has no other symptoms, such as glare, halos, ghost images, shadows, or starbursts.

Laser-based Study

Step 1: Studying Tomographic Risk Factors

1. *Validate the maps:* Qs is OK, there is no significant difference in pupil center coordinates between the two eyes ($X + X = -0.29 + 0.43 = +0.14$, $Y - Y = 0 - 0.20 = -0.20$), as

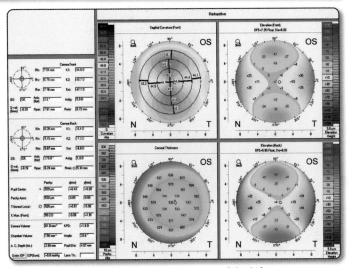

Fig. 8.2.2: The 4-composite map of the left eye.

shown in **Figure 8.2.3**, and there is no astigmatic disparity (**Table 8.2.2**). Therefore, the captures are accepted.

2. *Exclude factors of false positives and false negatives:* No factors exist.

3. *Apply the PS3 on the available data:* **Table 8.2.3** summarizes the study. Abnormal values are coded in orange for moderate-risk and red for high-risk factors. The table shows neither moderate-risk nor high-risk factors. **Table 8.2.4** represents the inter-eye asymmetry scoring.

4. Study the relative pachymetry map to rule out any previous corneal refractive surgery. The map is not available in this case.

5. Study pachymetric profiles to inspect for cornea guttata and Fuchs' dystrophy. The profiles are not available in this case.

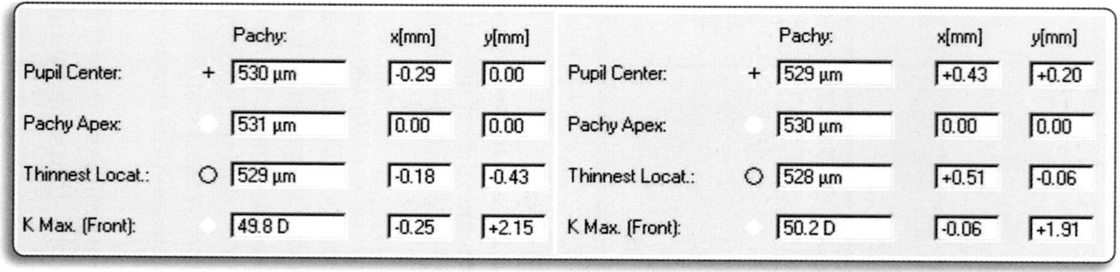

	Pachy.	x[mm]	y[mm]		Pachy.	x[mm]	y[mm]
Pupil Center: +	530 µm	-0.29	0.00	Pupil Center: +	529 µm	+0.43	+0.20
Pachy Apex: ●	531 µm	0.00	0.00	Pachy Apex: ●	530 µm	0.00	0.00
Thinnest Locat.: ○	529 µm	-0.18	-0.43	Thinnest Locat.: ○	528 µm	+0.51	-0.06
K Max. (Front): ◆	49.8 D	-0.25	+2.15	K Max. (Front): ◆	50.2 D	-0.06	+1.91

Fig. 8.2.3: Validating the maps by the pupil center coordinates.

Table 8.2.2: Astigmatic disparity.

	MA[a]	TA[a]	Disparity
OD	3.75 × 180°	3.80 × 003°	NO
OS	3.50 × 180°	4.00 × 002°	NO

(MA: manifest astigmatism; TA: tomographical astigmatism)
[a]Astigmatism is displayed in absolute value at the flat axis

Table 8.2.3: The practical subjective scoring system (PS3).

Parameters	OD	OS	Moderate	High
Ant. Km (D)	47	47.1	48–50	>50
TCT (µm)	529	528	470–500	<470
Inferior superior asymmetry (D)	S – I = 0.9	I – S = 0.2	I – S ≥ 1.5 S – I ≥ 2.5	NA
SRAX	0°	0°	NA	≥22°
Ant. Elevation (µm) @ TL	+3	+2	NA	≥8 emmetropia and myopia; ≥7 hyperopia and mixed astigmatism
Post. Elevation (µm) @ TL	+3	+4	NA	≥18 emmetropia and myopia; ≥28 hyperopia and mixed astigmatism
Pachymetry pattern	Concentric	Concentric	Dome, Droplet	Bell, Globus
Inter-eye asymmetry	Score 1[a]		Score 4	Score 5

(Ant. Km: mean K on the anterior corneal surface; TCT: thinnest corneal thickness; SRAX: skewed radial axis index; TL: thinnest location; NA: not available; SE: spherical aberration)
[a]See table 8.2.4

Table 8.2.4: Inter-eye asymmetry scoring.

Parameters	OD	OS	Score	Abnormal
Ant. Km (D)	47	47.1	0	≥0.3
Post. Km (D)	−6.7	−6.8	1	≥0.1
TCT (μm)	529	528	0	≥12
Ant. Elevation (μm) @ TL	+3	+2	0	≥2
Post. Elevation (μm) @ TL	+3	+4	0	≥5
Total			1	5

(Ant. Km: mean K on the anterior corneal surface; Post. Km: mean K on posterior corneal surface; TCT: thinnest corneal thickness; TL: thinnest location)

6. The patient has no symptoms, the CDVA = 1.0, and there is no irregularity in tomography. No need to study corneal wavefront.

Step 2: Considering Refractive Error Magnitude

1. The refractive error magnitude is within the range of correction in surface ablation and LASIK. Regarding SMILE, it is accepted according to the CE Mark, but it is contraindicated according to the FDA Approval because of high astigmatism.
2. The mesopic pupil is <7 mm in diameter.
3. **Table 8.2.5** shows the SE and TR for this case.
4. Since the magnitude of planned astigmatism is ≥1.50 D in both eyes, cyclotorsion compensation is recommended.
5. Recentration technique is recommended for two reasons, astigmatism in both eyes is ≥1.50 D, and the X coordinate of angle Kappa is >200 μm in the left eye; (−195 μm, 0 μm) in OD and (+215 μm, +100 μm) in OS. Holladay report is not

Table 8.2.5: Spherical equivalent (SE) and total refraction (TR).

	Sph (D)	Cyl (D)	SE (D)	TR (D)
OD	−2.50	−3.75	−4.38	−6.25
OS	−3.00	−3.50	−4.75	−6.50

(SE: spherical equivalent; TR: total refraction)

available in this case; therefore, angle Kappa coordinates are calculated by dividing pupil center coordinates by 2 (*see* **Fig. 8.2.3**).

Step 3: Calculations for Thickness and K-readings

In this case, thickness calculations will be done based on:
1. 6.5 mm OZ for all options.
2. 130 µm flap for LASIK.
3. 135 µm cap and 15 µm side cut for SMILE.

Tables 8.2.6 and 8.2.7 show calculations for PRK/surface ablation and LASIK/FemtoLASIK, respectively.

As shown in **Table 8.2.7**, the PTA is >40%, so LASIK/FemtoLASIK in not suitable. There are two solutions—either to reduce OZ diameter or to reduce flap thickness. Reducing the OZ is not recommended, especially with such high refractive error to avoid small efficient postoperative OZ, which is the leading cause of postoperative induced SA. The best solution is to reduce flap thickness. **Table 8.2.8** shows the PTA calculations for different flap thicknesses.

As shown in **Table 8.2.8**, to go for LASIK/FemtoLASIK, flap thickness should be ≤110 µm. It should be kept in mind that the standard deviation of flap thickness, even with Femtosecond laser, is ±18 µm, so it is recommended to go for 90 or 100 µm flap thickness.

Table 8.2.9 represents the calculations for SMILE.

Table 8.2.6: Thickness calculations for PRK/Surface ablation.

	TR (D)	CAD (µm)	Pre-op CCT (µm)	Post-op CCT (µm)	PRK
OD	−6.25	94	531	437	✓
OS	−6.50	98	530	432	✓

(TR: total refraction; CAD: central ablation depth; CCT: central corneal thickness

Table 8.2.7: Thickness calculations for LASIK/FemtoLASIK.

	TR (D)	CAD (µm)	Pre-op CCT (µm)	PTA	LASIK
OD	−6.25	94	531	42.18%	X
OS	−6.50	98	530	43.01%	X

(TR: total refraction; CAD: central ablation depth; CCT: central corneal thickness; PTA: percent tissue altered

Table 8.2.8: PTA calculations for LASIK/FemtoLASIK.

	CAD (µm)	Pre-op CCT (µm)	PTA			
			120 µm	110 µm	100 µm	90 µm
OD	94	531	40.3%	38.41%	36.53%	34.65%
OS	98	530	41.13%	39.24%	37.35%	35.47%

(CAD: central ablation depth; CCT: central corneal thickness; PTA: percent tissue altered)

Table 8.2.9: Thickness calculations for FemtoSMILE.

	TR (D)	Pre-op CCT (µm)	Lenticule (µm)	Bed (µm)	Post-op CCT (µm)	SMILE
OD	−6.25	531	111	285	420	✓
OS	−6.50	530	115	280	415	✓

(TR: total refraction; CCT: central corneal thickness)

Table 8.2.10 represents K-reading calculations for laser-based procedures.

Table 8.2.10: K-reading calculations.

	SE (D)	Pre-op ant. Km (D)	Change (D)	Post-op Ant. Km (D)	Laser-based
OD	−4.38	47	−3.5	43.5	✓
OS	−4.75	47.1	−3.8	43.3	✓

(SE: spherical equivalent; Ant. Km: mean K on the anterior corneal surface)

Step 4: Astigmatic Study

The TCRP is not available in this case. Therefore, the TA is calculated from the anterior and posterior surfaces. There is no astigmatic disparity in both eyes, as shown in **Table 8.2.1**. Probability No.2 applies here.

Step 5: Studying Both Eyes

Studying both eyes shows no inter-eye asymmetry (*see* **Table 8.2.4**), no ECDs, and no suspect of corneal pathologies.

Lens-based Study

Step 1: Study Tomography

In the laser-based study, tomography maps were validated, factors of false findings were excluded, ECDs were ruled out. Unfortunately, the relative pachymetry map and the pachymetry profiles are not available in this case.

Step 2: Study Parameters

1. *In PIOL Implantation:*
   - *AC parameters:* As shown in **Figure 8.2.4**, the internal ACD is 3.09 mm in OD and 2.99 mm in OS. ACA is 34° in OD and 33.6° in OS. ACV is 153 mm^3 in OD and 155 mm^3 in OS. All values are suitable for both types of PIOL implantation.

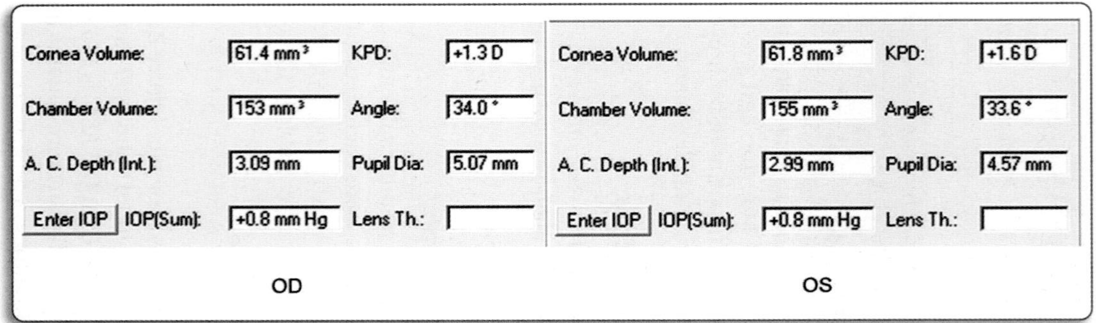

Fig. 8.2.4: Anterior chamber parameters.

OD			
Cornea Volume:	61.4 mm³	KPD:	+1.3 D
Chamber Volume:	153 mm³	Angle:	34.0 °
A. C. Depth (Int.):	3.09 mm	Pupil Dia:	5.07 mm
Enter IOP IOP(Sum):	+0.8 mm Hg	Lens Th.:	

OS			
Cornea Volume:	61.8 mm³	KPD:	+1.6 D
Chamber Volume:	155 mm³	Angle:	33.6 °
A. C. Depth (Int.):	2.99 mm	Pupil Dia:	4.57 mm
Enter IOP IOP(Sum):	+0.8 mm Hg	Lens Th.:	

- *HWTW diameter:* Holladay report is not available in this case. However, HWTW is more accurately measured by optical devices.
- The mesopic pupil is <7 mm.
- Consider MA rather than tomographic astigmatism.

2. *CLE and Monofocal IOL Implantation:*
   - ACD is within the normal range in both eyes, so no special considerations in IOL calculations.
   - The posterior astigmatism is >0.5 D in both eyes, as shown in the 4-composite maps. This affects the measurement of toric IOL if the true TCRP astigmatism is not considered. Consider the SIA and incision type, shape, size, and location.
   - *HWTW diameter:* If the diameter is within the normal range, the IOL can be implanted safely; otherwise, a customized haptic-to-haptic diameter is required.
   - Consider TCRP astigmatism rather than tomographic astigmatism.

3. *CLE and Premium IOL Implantation:*
   - Mesopic pupil diameter is 5.07 mm in OD and 4.57 mm in OS (*see* **Fig. 8.2.4**). It is within the accepted range. However, it is more accurately measured by an infrared-based pupillometer.
   - ACD is within the normal range in both eyes, so no special considerations in IOL calculations.
   - The posterior astigmatism is >0.5 D in both eyes. That affects the measurement of the premium IOL if the true TCRP astigmatism is not considered.
   - If a non-toric premium IOL is planned, the TCRP astigmatism should be <0.75 D. Unfortunately, the TCRP is not available, but we can have an idea by calculating the TA. The TA is >0.75 in both eyes, as shown in **Table 8.2.2.** Therefore, non-toric premium

IOL is contraindicated unless the astigmatism is treated or a toric-premium IOL is planned. Consider the SIA and incision type, shape, size, and location.

- *HWTW diameter:* If the diameter is within the normal range, the IOL can be implanted safely; otherwise, a customized haptic-to-haptic diameter is needed.
- *Angle kappa:* Based on pupil center coordinates, angle kappa is around (–195 µm, 0 µm) in OD and (+215 µm, +100 µm) in OS. It is within the accepted range.
- Consider TCRP astigmatism rather than tomographic astigmatism.

Step 3: Study Corneal Wavefront

1. *In PIOL implantation:*
   - *Corneal regularity:* Although the anterior sagittal curvature map is regular and at low risk (no significant superior, inferior difference and no significant SRAX), corneal wavefront shows high HOAs RMS (>0.35 µm), mainly on account of the SA. **Figures 8.2.5 and 8.2.6** represent corneal wavefront for OD and OS, respectively. Despite this high HOAs RMS, the patient is asymptomatic. Therefore, good results are expected.
2. *CLE and Monofocal IOL implantation:*
   - The total RMS is >0.35 µm on account of SA. As shown in **Figures 8.2.4 and 8.2.5**, the SA is +ve and >0.35 µm. Following the PSIS algorithm (*see* **Fig. 2.47**), the choice of IOL depends on patient's demands. If the image quality is critical, an aspheric IOL with –ve SA is recommended; –0.27 type in OD and –0.20 type in OS to achieve the target. If the DOF is critical, an aspheric IOL with zero-SA is recommended.

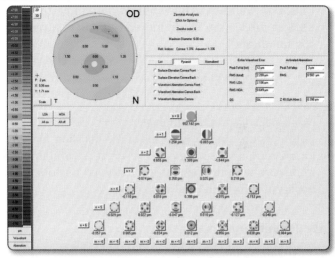

Fig. 8.2.5: Corneal wavefront of the right eye.

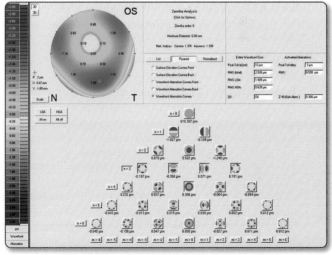

Fig. 8.2.6: Corneal wavefront of the left eye.

3. *CLE and Premium IOL Implantation:* Since the total RMS is >0.35 μm, this type of refractive surgery is contraindicated.

Step 4: Study Both Eyes

1. No ECDs in both eyes.
2. No suspect of corneal pathologies.
3. Both eyes are similar in terms of the decision for lens-based refractive surgery. However, it is fundamental to discuss with the patient the expected postoperative quality of vision and DOF in each eye.

Case 2 Summary

Based on corneal tomography:

- All types of laser-based refractive surgery are suitable. **Table 8.2.11** represents the recommendations.
- PIOL implantation is suitable with no special precautions.
- CLE and monofocal IOL implantation is suitable, but an aspheric IOL with zero-SA is recommended.
- CLE and premium IOL implantation is contraindicated.

Table 8.2.11: Recommendations for laser-based refractive surgery.

	PRK	LASIK[a]	SMILE[b]	OZ (mm)	Cyclotorsion compensation	Recentration
OD	✓	✓	✓ (CE Mark)	6.5	✓	Not necessary
OS	✓	✓	✓ (CE Mark)	6.5	✓	✓

(OZ: optical zone)
[a]Flap ≤ 100 μm
[b]Cap = 135 μm and side cut = 15 μm

■ CASE 3

A 31-year-old female visiting for refractive surgery. Her subjective refraction is shown in **Table 8.3.1,** and her 4-composite refractive maps are shown in **Figures 8.3.1 and 8.3.2**. The patient has some halos and starbursts at night.

Laser-based Study

Step 1: Studying Tomographic Risk Factors

1. *Validate the maps:* Qs is OK, but there is an inter-eye difference in X coordinate of pupil center ($X + X = -0.24$ mm $= -240$ μm > 200) as shown in **Figure 8.3.3**. **Figures 8.3.4 and 8.3.5** are power distribution for OD and OS, respectively. The TCRP astigmatism at 3 mm ring/apex is compared with the MA. There is astigmatic disparity in OD **(Table 8.3.2)**.

    Based on the above, the captures should be repeated, and factors of false findings should be ruled out. The first thing to come to mind is misalignment that can explain the SRAX and astigmatic disparity in OD. All factors of false findings were ruled out, and the patient was taught how to fixate properly during the captures. The captures were repeated and stayed the same. Therefore, the captures with the *least* inter-eye difference in pupil center coordinates were considered, and this case is considered as a real inter-eye asymmetry and will be studied accordingly.

Table 8.3.1: Subjective refraction.

	Sph (D)	Cyl (D)	Axis	CDVA
OD	+0.75	−2.75	170°	1.0
OS	+1.00	−2.00	005°	1.0

(CDVA: corrected distance visual acuity measured in decimal)

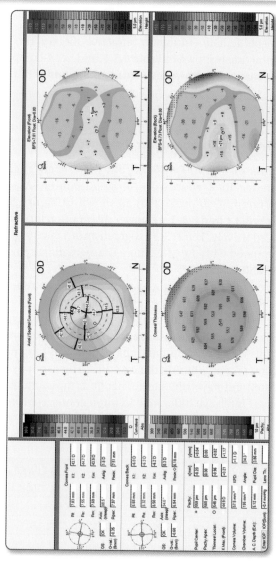

Fig. 8.3.1: The 4-composite map of the right eye.

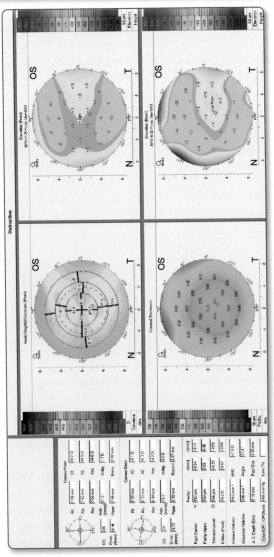

Fig. 8.3.2: The 4-composite map of the left eye.

	Pachy:	x[mm]	y[mm]		Pachy:	x[mm]	y[mm]
Pupil Center:	+ 559 μm	-0.20	+0.04	Pupil Center:	+ 563 μm	-0.04	-0.11
Pachy Apex:	· 560 μm	0.00	0.00	Pachy Apex:	· 564 μm	0.00	0.00
Thinnest Locat.:	O 548 μm	-0.96	-0.82	Thinnest Locat.:	O 556 μm	+0.33	-0.99
K Max. (Front):	44.9 D	+0.21	+1.17	K Max. (Front):	45.2 D	-0.07	-0.99
	OD				OS		

Fig. 8.3.3: Validating the maps by the pupil center coordinates.

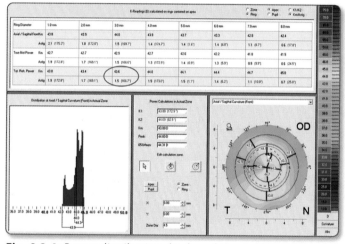

Fig. 8.3.4: Power distribution display of the right eye. The true corneal astigmatism by the total corneal refractive power (TCRP) at 3 mm ring/apex (red ellipse).

2. Exclude factors of false positives and false negatives: no factors exist.

3. The patient has other complimentary maps and profiles. **Figures 8.3.6 and 8.3.7** are pachymetric profiles for OD and OS, respectively. The profiles are within the normal range, although slightly flat. **Figures 8.3.8 and 8.3.9** represent Belin-Ambrosio Display (BAD) for OD and OS,

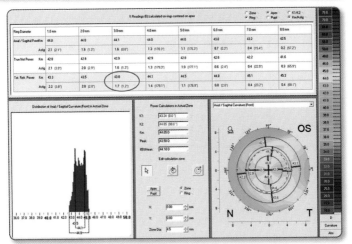

Fig. 8.3.5: Power distribution display of the left eye. The true corneal astigmatism by the total corneal refractive power (TCRP) at 3 mm ring/apex (red ellipse).

Table 8.3.2: Astigmatic disparity.			
	MAª	TAª	Disparity
OD	2.75 × 170°	1.50 × 167°	YES
OS	2.00 × 005°	1.70 × 001°	NO

(MA: manifest astigmatism; TA: tomographical astigmatism)
ªAstigmatism is displayed in absolute value at the flat axis.

respectively. The BAD is normal in both eyes. **Figures 8.3.10 and 8.3.11** are relative pachymetric maps for OD and OS, respectively. They are within the normal range.

4. *Apply the PS3 on the available data:* **Table 8.3.3** summarizes the study. Abnormal values are coded in orange for moderate-risk and red for high-risk factors. **Table 8.3.4** represents the inter-eye asymmetry scoring.

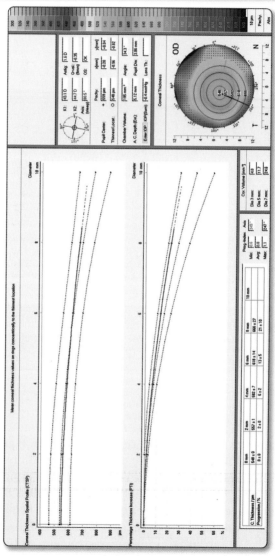

Fig. 8.3.6: Corneal thickness profiles of the right eye.

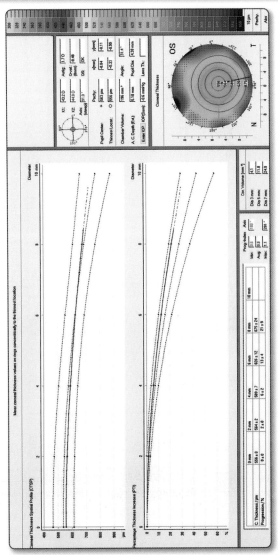

Fig. 8.3.7: Corneal thickness profiles of the left eye.

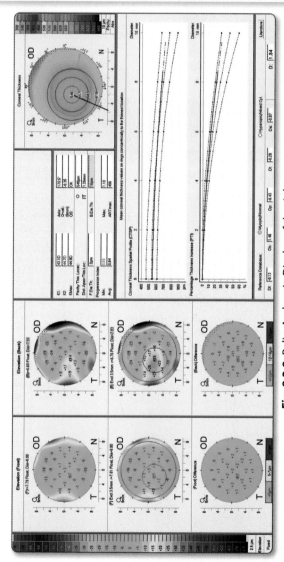

Fig. 8.3.8: Belin-Ambrosio Display of the right eye.

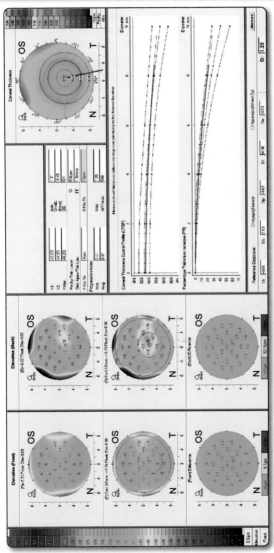

Fig. 8.3.9: Belin-Ambrosio Display of the left eye.

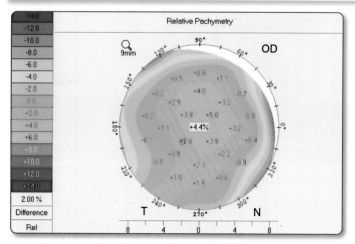

Fig. 8.3.10: The relative pachymetry map of the right eye.

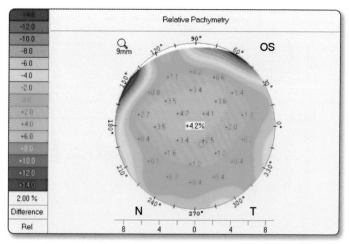

Fig. 8.3.11: The relative pachymetry map of the left eye.

Table 8.3.3: The practical subjective scoring system (PS3).

Parameters	OD	OS	Moderate	High
Ant. Km (D)	43.9	44	48–50	>50
TCT (µm)	548	556	470–500	<470
Inferior superior asymmetry (D)	I – S = 0.4	S – I = 0.3	I – S ≥ 1.5 S – I ≥ 2.5	NA
SRAX	> 22°	0°	NA	≥22°
Ant. Elevation (µm) @ TL	+3	+1	NA	≥8 emmetropia and myopia; ≥7 hyperopia and mixed astigmatism
Post. Elevation (µm) @ TL	+17	+15	NA	≥18 emmetropia and myopia; ≥28 hyperopia and mixed astigmatism
Pachymetry pattern	Dome	Dome	Dome, Droplet	Bell, Globus
Pachymetric Profiles	Normal	Normal	S after 6; avg. ≥ 1.2	Quick slope; S before 6 mm; Inverted
Relative Pachymetry Maps	Normal	Normal	< –8%	NA
Inter-eye asymmetry	Score 1[a]		Score 4	Score 5

(Ant. Km: mean K on the anterior corneal surface; TCT: thinnest corneal thickness; SRAX: skewed radial axis index; TL: thinnest location; NA: not available; SE: spherical aberration)
[a]See table 8.3.4

Based on the PS3, there is one high-risk factor in OD and one moderate-risk factor in each eye. According to the author's opinion, such a case is a contraindication for laser-based refractive surgery.

Table 8.3.4: Inter-eye asymmetry scoring.

Parameters	OD	OS	Score	Abnormal
Ant. Km (D)	43.9	44	0	≥0.3
Post. Km (D)	−6.2	−6.2	0	≥0.1
TCT (μm)	548	556	0	≥12
Ant. Elevation (μm) @ TL	+3	+1	1	≥2
Post. Elevation (μm) @ TL	+17	+15	0	≥5
Total			1	5

(Ant. Km: mean K on the anterior corneal surface; Post. Km: mean K on posterior corneal surface; TCT: thinnest corneal thickness; TL: thinnest location)

Lens-based Study

Step 1: Study Tomography

In the laser-based study, tomography maps were validated, factors of false findings were excluded, ECDs were ruled out. Based on the pachymetry profiles, there is no suspect of guttata or Fuchs' dystrophy. Based on the relative pachymetry maps, there is no suspect of previous corneal surgeries.

Step 2: Study Parameters

1. *In PIOL Implantation:*
   - *AC parameters:* As shown in **Figure 8.3.12**, the ACD is measured externally (including corneal thickness) rather than internally. Therefore, the internal ACD is 5.12 – 0.548 (CCT) = 4.572 mm in OD and 5.12 – 0.556 (CCT) = 4.564 mm in OS. That is a deep AC in both eyes. The ACA is 34.3° in OD and 31.4° in OS. The ACV is 195 mm³ in OD and 196 mm³ in OS. All values are suitable for both types of PIOL implantation.

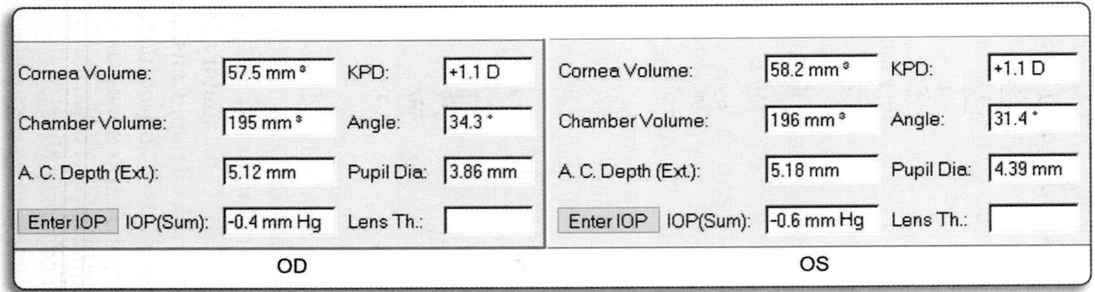

Fig. 8.3.12: Anterior chamber parameters.

- *HWTW diameter:* **Figures 8.3.13 and 8.3.14** represent Holladay report in OD and OS, respectively. HWTW is 12.1 mm in both eyes (red ellipse). It is within the normal range. However, HWTW is more accurately measured by optical devices.
- The mesopic pupil is <7 mm.
- Consider MA rather than tomographic astigmatism.

2. *Clear Lens Extraction (CLE) and Monofocal IOL Implantation:*
   - *ACD:* The AC is relatively deep in both eyes, so special formulas are needed for IOL calculations.
   - The posterior astigmatism is <0.5 D in both eyes. However, the TCRP is mandatory in the formulas of toric IOL calculation. Consider the SIA and incision type, shape, size, and location.
   - *HWTW diameter:* Since it is within the normal range, the standard haptic-to-haptic IOL size can be implanted safely in the bag.
   - Consider TCRP astigmatism rather than MA.

3. *CLE and Premium IOL Implantation:*
   - Mesopic pupil diameter is 3.86 mm in OD and 4.39 mm in OS (*see Fig. 8.3.12*). It is within the accepted range. However, it is more accurately measured by an infrared-based pupillometer.
   - *ACD:* The AC is relatively deep in both eyes, so special formulas are needed for IOL calculations.
   - The posterior astigmatism is <0.5 D in both eyes. However, the TCRP is mandatory in the formulas of premium IOL calculation. Consider the SIA and incision type, shape, size, and location.
   - A non-toric premium IOL is contraindicated because the TCRP astigmatism is >0.75.
   - *HWTW diameter:* Since it is within the normal range, the IOL can be implanted safely in the bag.

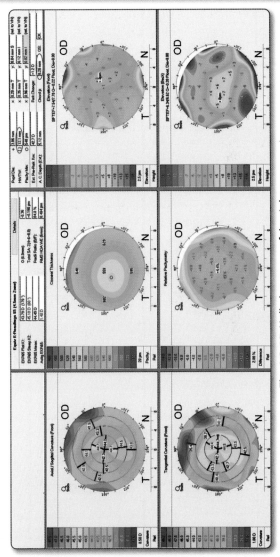

Fig. 8.3.13: Holladay report of the right eye.

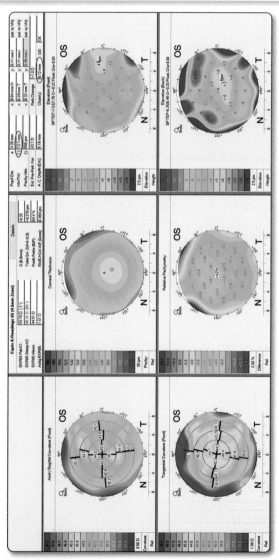

Fig. 8.3.14: Holladay report of the left eye.

- *Angle kappa:* Based on the Holladay report, chord μ is 0.20 mm in OD and 0.12 mm in OS. It is within the accepted range.
- Consider TCRP astgmatism rather than MA.

Step 3: Study Corneal Wavefront

1. *PIOL Implantation:* **Figures 8.3.15 and 8.3.16** represent corneal wavefront for OD and OS, respectively. The total RMS in OD is 0.405 μm, which is abnormal on account of horizontal trefoil and SA. The total RMS in OS is 0.37 μm, which is abnormal on account of SA. That explains the halos and starbursts at night. Such symptoms usually persist after PIOL implantation and should be discussed with the patient.

2. *CLE and Monofocal IOL Implantation:*
   - A toric IOL should be implanted.
   - The total RMS is >0.35 μm in both eyes. Extracting the crystalline lens changes the situation of the ocular HOAs and may worsen the symptoms and affect the quality of postoperative visual acuity.
   - In OD, the total RMS is high on account of horizontal trefoil and SA. According to the PSIS algorithm, an aspheric IOL with zero-SA is recommended (*see* **Fig. 2.44**).
   - In OS, the total RMS is high on account of SA. The PSIS algorithm can be applied (*see* **Fig. 2.47**). Since the cornea is virgin and the SA is +ve, an aspheric IOL with −0.27 SA is implanted, if the image quality is critical to the patient; otherwise, an aspheric IOL with zero-SA is implanted, if DOF is preferred.

3. *CLE and Premium IOL Implantation:* Since the total RMS is > 0.35 μm, this type of refractive surgery is contraindicated.

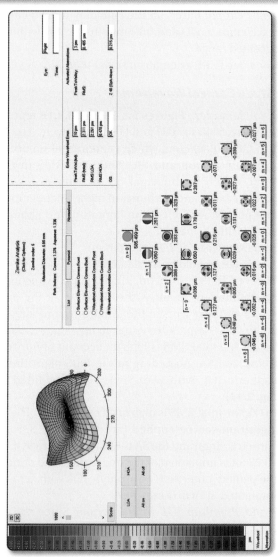

Fig. 8.3.15: Corneal wavefront. Zernike analysis of the right eye.

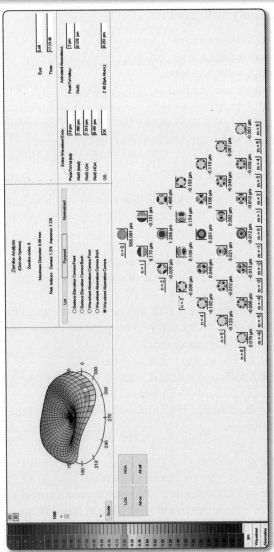

Fig. 8.3.16: Corneal wavefront. Zernike analysis of the left eye.

Step 4: Study Both Eyes

1. No ECDs in both eyes.
2. No suspect of corneal pathologies because factors of false findings were excluded.
3. Both eyes are similar in terms of the decision for lens-based refractive surgery. However, it is fundamental to discuss with the patient the expected postoperative quality of vision and DOF in each eye.

Case 3 Summary

Based on Corneal Tomography

- All types of laser-based refractive surgery are not suitable for both eyes.
- Toric PIOL implantation is suitable for both eyes. The postoperative symptoms should be discussed with the patient.
- CLE and monofocal IOL implantation are possible for both eyes, but the quality of postoperative vision will most probably not be optimum:
  - *OD:* A toric aspheric IOL with zero-SA.
  - *OS:* A toric aspheric IOL with –0.27 SA for better image quality, or zero-SA for better DOF.
- CLE and premium IOL implantation are contraindicated in both eyes.

■ CASE 4

A 55-year-old male visiting for vision correction and asking about presbyopia treatment. The patient has a foggy vision in daylight. **Table 8.4.1** shows his subjective refraction. Slit-lamp biomicroscopy revealed posterior subcapsular cataract

Table 8.4.1: Subjective refraction.

	Sph (D)	Cyl (D)	Axis	CDVA	Add	CNVA
OD	+2.00	−2.50	20°	0.7	+2.25	0.8
OS	+1.00	−2.75	005°	0.6	+2.25	0.8

(CDVA: corrected distance visual acuity measured in decimal; CNVA: corrected near visual acuity measured in decimal)

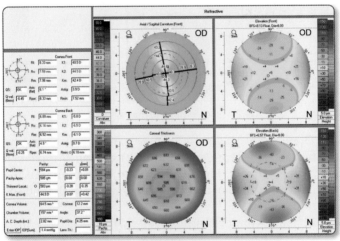

Fig. 8.4.1: The 4-composite map of the right eye.

in both eyes. This is a case of cataract and will be studied based on tomography. All other investigations were normal.

Figures 8.4.1 and 8.4.2 are the 4-composite refractive maps for OD and OS, respectively.

Step 1: Study Tomography

1. *Validate the maps:* Qs is OK, and there is no significant difference in pupil center coordinates between the two eyes ($X + X = -190$ μm < 200), as shown in **Figure 8.4.3**.

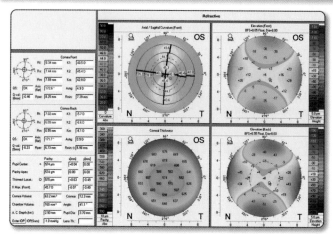

Fig. 8.4.2: The 4-composite map of the left eye.

There is an astigmatic disparity that persists despite repeating the captures **(Table 8.4.2)** and can be explained by the cataract. **Figures 8.4.4 and 8.4.5** represent the power distribution and TCRP astigmatism in OD and OS, respectively.

2. Exclude factors of false positives and false negatives. Apart from the cataract, no factors exist.

3. Study tomography systematically, check regularity, and rule out ECDs. The patient has all complimentary maps, including pachymetric profiles **(Figs. 8.4.6 and 8.4.7)**, BAD **(Figs. 8.4.8 and 8.4.9)**, and the relative pachymetry maps **(Figs. 8.4.10 and 8.4.11)**. **Tables 8.4.3 and 8.3.4** represent the PS3 and inter-eye asymmetry study, respectively. No irregularity and no asymmetry exist.

4. Study the relative pachymetry map to rule out any previous corneal refractive surgery. The maps are normal and do not show any pattern of a previous corneal refractive surgery.

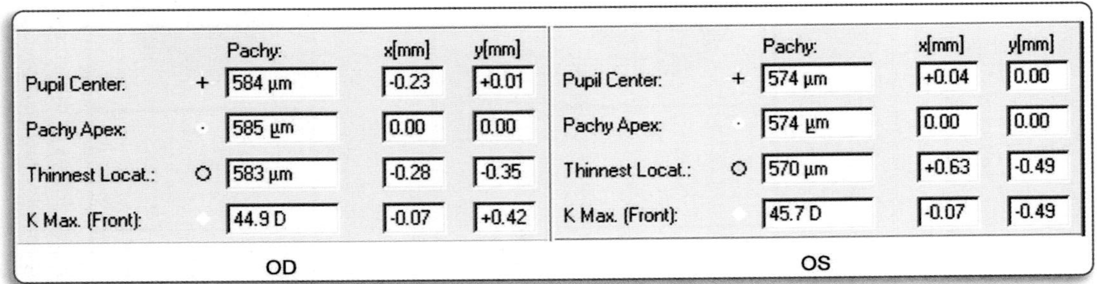

OD

Pupil Center:	Pachy:	+	584 µm	x[mm]	-0.23	y[mm]	+0.01
Pachy Apex:		·	585 µm		0.00		0.00
Thinnest Locat.:		○	583 µm		-0.28		-0.35
K Max. (Front):		◆	44.9 D		-0.07		+0.42

OS

Pupil Center:	Pachy:	+	574 µm	x[mm]	+0.04	y[mm]	0.00
Pachy Apex:		·	574 µm		0.00		0.00
Thinnest Locat.:		○	570 µm		+0.63		-0.49
K Max. (Front):		◆	45.7 D		-0.07		-0.49

Fig. 8.4.3: Validating the maps by the pupil center coordinates.

Table 8.4.2: Astigmatic disparity.			
	MA[a]	*TA*[a]	*Disparity*
OD	$2.50 \times 20°$	$3.40 \times 6°$	YES
OS	$2.75 \times 005°$	$4.70 \times 173°$	YES

(MA: manifest astigmatism; TA: tomographical astigmatism)
[a]Astigmatism is displayed in absolute value at the flat axis.

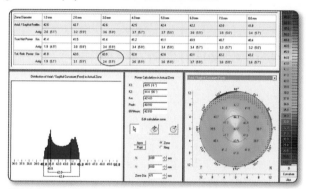

Fig. 8.4.4: Power distribution display of the right eye. The true corneal astigmatism by the total corneal refractive power (TCRP) at 3 mm ring/apex (red ellipse).

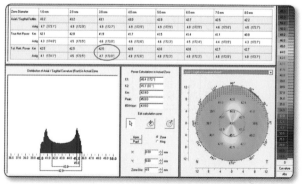

Fig. 8.4.5: Power distribution display of the left eye. The true corneal astigmatism by the total corneal refractive power (TCRP) at 3 mm ring/apex (red ellipse).

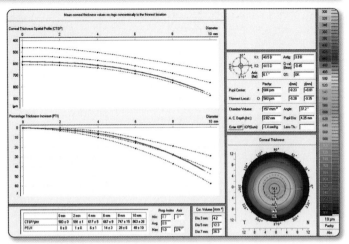

Fig. 8.4.6: Corneal thickness profiles of the right eye.

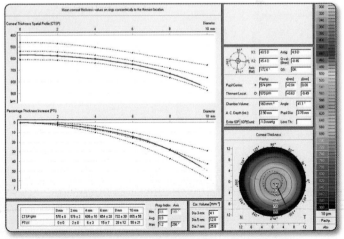

Fig. 8.4.7: Corneal thickness profiles of the left eye.

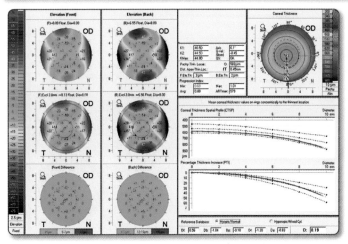

Fig. 8.4.8: Belin-Ambrosio Display of the right eye.

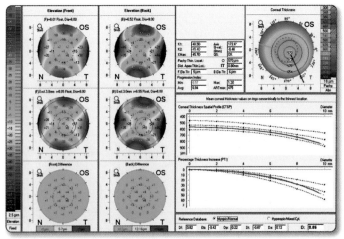

Fig. 8.4.9: Belin-Ambrosio Display of the left eye.

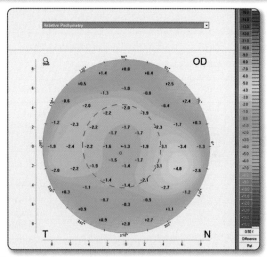

Fig. 8.4.10: The relative pachymetry map of the right eye.

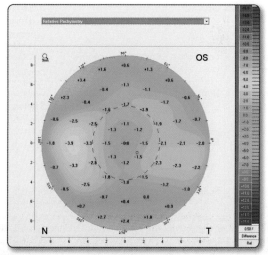

Fig. 8.4.11: The relative pachymetry map of the left eye.

Table 8.4.3: The Practical Subjective Scoring System (PS3).

Parameters	OD	OS	Moderate	High
Ant. Km (D)	42.4	42.8	48–50	>50
TCT (μm)	583	570	470–500	<470
Inferior superior asymmetry (D)	S – I = 0.6	I – S = 0	I – S ≥ 1.5 S – I ≥ 2.5	NA
SRAX	0°	0°	NA	≥22°
Ant. Elevation (μm) @ TL	+5	+6	NA	≥8 emmetropia and myopia; ≥7 hyperopia and mixed astigmatism
Post. Elevation (μm) @ TL	+4	+8	NA	≥18 emmetropia and myopia; ≥28 hyperopia and mixed astigmatism
Pachymetry pattern	Concentric	Concentric	Dome, Droplet	Bell, Globus
Pachymetric Profiles	Normal	Normal	S after 6; avg. ≥1.2	Quick slope; S before 6 mm; Inverted
Relative Pachymetry Maps	Normal	Normal	< –8%	NA
Inter-eye asymmetry	Score 2[a]		Score 4	Score 5

(Ant. Km: mean K on the anterior corneal surface; TCT: thinnest corneal thickness; SRAX: skewed radial axis index; TL: thinnest location; NA: not available; SE: spherical aberration)
[a]See table 8.4.4

Table 8.4.4: Inter-eye asymmetry scoring.

Parameters	OD	OS	Score	Abnormal
Ant. Km (D)	42.4	42.8	1	≥0.3
Post. Km (D)	–6.1	–6.1	0	≥0.1
TCT (µm)	583	570	1	≥12
Ant. Elevation (µm) @ TL	+5	+6	0	≥2
Post. Elevation (µm) @ TL	+4	+8	0	≥5
Total			2	5

(Ant. Km: mean K on the anterior corneal surface; Post. Km: mean K on posterior corneal surface; TCT: thinnest corneal thickness; TL: thinnest location)

5. Study pachymetric profiles to exclude cornea guttata and Fuchs' dystrophy. As shown in **Figures 8.4.6 and 8.4.7**, the pachymetric profiles are not flat, and therefore, there is no *tomographic* sign of the two diseases. However, they can be excluded only by specular microscopy.

Step 2: Study Parameters

1. *Mesopic pupil size:* It is 4.25 mm in OD and 3.70 mm in OS. No contraindication for premium IOL implantation. However, it is more accurately measured by an infrared-based pupillometer.
2. *ACD:* It is within the normal range in both eyes, 2.82 mm in OD and 2.90 mm in OS, so no special considerations.
3. *TCRP astigmatism and posterior astigmatism:* The astigmatism is high, so a toric IOL is recommended. The posterior astigmatism is >0.5 D in both eyes. However, TCRP astigmatism is mandatory for toric IOL calculation. Consider the SIA and incision type, shape, size, and location.

4. If astigmatic keratotomy (AK) or limbal-relaxing incisions (LRIs) are planned, TCRP is mandatory and special algorithms are available.

5. *Angle kappa:* **Figures 8.4.12 and 8.4.13** represent the Holladay report in OD and OS, respectively. Unfortunately, this report does not show the chord μ because it is in the old version. Therefore, based on *X* and *Y* pupil center coordinates, angle kappa is insignificant and no contraindication for premium IOL implantation.

6. *HWTW:* As mentioned above, the Holladay report is in the old version and does not show HWTW. However, it is more accurately measured by optical devices. If it is within the normal range, there are no special considerations for the haptic-to-haptic diameter.

Step 4: Study Corneal Wavefront

Figures 8.4.14 and **8.4.15** are Zernike analysis for OD and OS, respectively. The total RMS is < 0.35 μm in both eyes. Therefore, no contraindication for premium IOL implantation. The SA is close to +0.1 μm in both eyes. Therefore, according to PSIS algorithm **(Fig. 2.44)**, if quality of vision is preferred, an aspheric IOL with zero-SA is recommended; otherwise, a premium IOL is recommended if DOF is preferred.

Step 4: Study Both Eyes

1. No ECDs.
2. No corneal irregularities and no corneal pathologies.
   IOL type should be discussed based on patient's demands.
3. This case is a bilateral cataract.
4. IOL type should be discussed based on patient's demands.

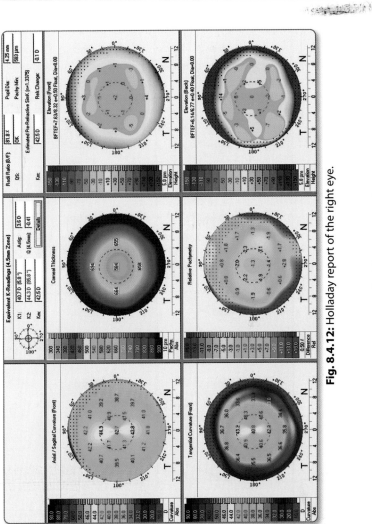

Fig. 8.4.12: Holladay report of the right eye.

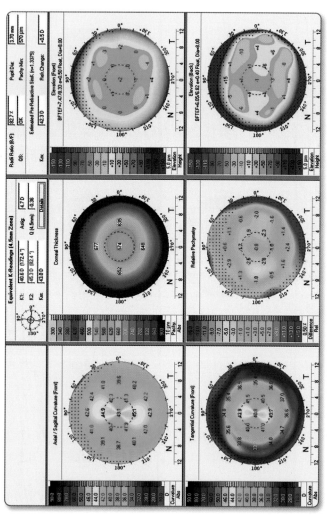

Fig. 8.4.13: Holladay report of the left eye.

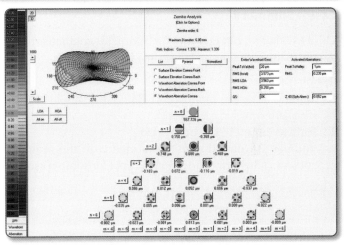

Fig. 8.4.14: Corneal wavefront. Zernike analysis of the right eye.

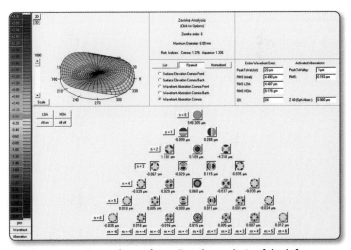

Fig. 8.4.15: Corneal wavefront. Zernike analysis of the left eye.

Case 4 Summary

This is a bilateral cataract with high corneal astigmatism. The patient is interested in spectacle-free for reading.

Options of IOLs:

1. Monovision/mini-monovision. Both IOLs should be toric with zero-SA.
2. Toric premium IOL in both eyes.
3. Additive AK or LRI can be planned with the previous options, if the toric type is not possible for some reason.

Bibliography

1. Abad JC, Rubinfeld RS, Valle MD, Belin MW, Kurstin JM. Vertical D: a novel topographic in some keratoconus suspects. Ophthalmology. 2007;114(5):1020-6.

2. Alfonso JF, Fernández-Vega L, Lisa C, Fernandes P, Jorge J, Montés Micó R. Central vault after phakic intraocular lens implantation: correlation with anterior chamber depth, white-to-white distance, spherical equivalent, and patient age. J Cataract Refract Surg. 2012;38(1):46-53.

3. Alio JL, and Shabayek MH. Corneal high order aberrations: a method to grade keratoconus. J Refract Surg. 2006;22:539-45.

4. Ambrosio Jr R, de Oliveira Ramos IC, Luz A, et al. In: Belin MW, Khachikian SS and Ambrosio Jr R (Eds). Comprehensive Pachymetric Evaluation in Elevation Based Corneal Tomography, 2nd edn. Jaypee-Highlights Medical Publisher, Inc.; 2012 .pp. 25-45.

5. Amesbury EC, Miller KM. Correction of astigmatism at the time of cataract surgery. Curr Opin Ophthalmol. 2009;20(1):19-24.

6. Amsler M. The "forme fruste" of keratoconus (in German). Wien Klin Wochenschr. 1961;73:842-3.

7. Arba-Mosquera S, Merayo-Lloves J, de Ortueta D. Clinical Effects of Pure Cyclotorsional Errors during Refractive Surgery. Invest Ophthalmology & Visual Science. 2008;49:4828-36.

8. Arba-Mosquera S, Verma S, McAlinden C. Centration axis in refractive surgery. Eye Vis (Lond). 2015;2:4. Published 2015 Feb 24. doi:10.1186/s40662-015-0014-6.

9. Arbelaez MC, Versaci F, Vestri G, et al. Use of a support vector machine for keratoconus and subclinical keratoconus detection by topographic and tomographic data. Ophthalmology. 2012;119(11):2231-8.

10. Armitage JA, Bruce AS, Philips AJ, Lindsay RG. Morphological variants in keratoconus: anatomical observation or aetiologically significant?. Aust NZJ Ophthalmol. 1998;26 (Suppl 1):S68-70.

11. Azar DT, Gatinel D. Refractive Surgery, 2nd edn. Philadelphia: Mosby Elsevier; 2007 .pp. 397-463.

12. Baikoff G, Bourgeon G, Jodai HJ, Fontaine A, Lellis FV, Trinquet L. Pigment dispersion and Artisan implants: crystalline lens rise as a safety criterion [article in French]. J Fr Ophtalmol. 2005;28:590-7.

13. Baillif S, Garweg JG, Grange JD, Burillon C, Kodjikian L. Keratoglobus: review of the literature. J Fr Ophthalmol. 2005; 28:1145-9.

14. Bayramlar H, Daglioglu MC, Borazan M. Limbal relaxing incisions for primary mixed astigmatism and mixed astigmatism after cataract surgery. J Cataract Refract Surg. 2003;29(4):723-8.

15. Belin MW, Ambrosio Jr R, Khachikian SS. Keratoconus/ectasia detection with a modified (enhanced) reference surface. In: Belin MW, Khachikian SS and Ambrosio Jr. R (Eds). Elevation Based Corneal Tomography, 2nd edn. Jaypee-Highlights Medical Publisher, Inc.; 2012 .pp. 93-104.

16. Belin MW, and Khachikian SS. Keratoconus: It's hard to define but. . . Am J Ophthalmol. 2007;43(3):500-3.

17. Belin MW, Asota IM, Ambrosio Jr R, Khachikian SS. What's in a name of: keratoconus, pellucid marginal degeneration, and related thinning disorders. Am J Ophthalmol. 2011;152:157-62.

18. Belin MW, Khachikian SS, Ambrosio Jr R. Understanding elevation based topography: how elevation data is displayed. In: Belin MW, Khachikian SS, Ambrosio Jr R (Eds). Elevation Based Corneal Tomography, 2nd edn. Jaypee-Highlights Medical Publisher, Inc.; 2012 .pp. 25-45.

19. Belin MW, Khachikian SS, and Ambrosio Jr. R. Suggested set-up and screening guidelines. In: Belin MW, Khachikian SS, Ambrosio Jr R (Eds). Elevation Based Corneal Tomography, 2nd edn. Jaypee-Highlights Medical Publisher, Inc.; 2012 .pp. 57-69.

20. Belin MW, Kim JT, Zloty P, Ambrosio R Jr. Simplified nomenclature for describing keratoconus. Int J Kerat Ect Cor Dis. 2012;1(1):31-5.

21. Benedetti S, Casamenti V, Benedetti M. Long-term endothelial changes in phakic eyes after Artisan intraocular lens implantation to correct myopia: five-year study. J Cataract Refract Surg. 2007;33:784-90.

22. Benes P, Synek S, and Petrova S. Corneal shape and eccentricity in population. Coll Antropol. 2013; (Suppl 1):117-20.

23. Binder PS, Trattler WB. Evaluation of a risk factor scoring system for corneal ectasia after LASIK in eyes with normal topography. J Refract Surg. 2010;26(4):241-50.

24. Bogan SJ, Waring GO III, Ibrahim O, Drews C, Curtis L. Classification of normal corneal topography based on computer-assisted videokeratography. Arch Ophthalmol. 1990;108(7): 945-9.

25. Bourne WM, Nelson LR, Hodge DO. Central corneal endothelial changes over a ten-year period. Invest Ophthalmol Vis Sci. 1997;38:779-82.

26. Boxer Wachler BS, Huynh VN, El-Shiaty, AF, Goldberg D. Evaluation of corneal functional optical zone after laser in situ keratomileusis. J Cataract Refract Surg. 2002;28:948-53.

27. Braga-Mele R, Chang D, Dewey S, Foster G, Henderson BN, Hill W, et al. Multifocal intraocular lenses: relative indications and contraindications for implantation. J Cataract Refract Surg. 2014;40:313-22.

28. Buhren J, Kook D, Yoon G, Kohnen T. Detection of subclinical keratoconus by using corneal anterior and posterior surface aberrations and thickness spatial profiles. Invest Ophthalmol Vis Sci. 2010;51:3424-32

29. Buhren J, Kuhne C, Kohnen T. Defining subclinical keratoconus using corneal first-surface higher-order aberrations. Am J Ophthalmol. 2007;143:381-9.

30. Bühren J, Kühne C, Kohnen T. Influence of pupil and optical zone diameter on higher-order aberrations after wavefront-guided myopic LASIK. J Cataract Refract Surg. 2005;31(12):2272-80.

31. Buhren J, Kuhne C, Kohnen T. Wavefront analysis for the diagnosis of subclinical keratoconus (in German). Ophthalmologe. 2006;103:783-90.

32. Calossi A. Corneal asphericity and spherical aberration. J Refract Surg. 2007;23:505-14.

33. Cameron JA, Al-Rajhi AA, Badr IA. Corneal ectasia in vernal keratoconjunctivitis. Ophthalmology. 1989;96(11):1615-23.

34. Chan A, Manche EE. Effect of Preoperative Pupil Size on Quality of Vision after Wavefront-Guided LASIK. Ophthalmology. 2011;118(4):736-41.

35. Chaudhry IA, El Danasoury MA. Phakic intraocular lenses. Saudi J Ophthalmol. 2013;27(4):231-3.

36. Chow SSW, Chow LLW, Lee CZ, Chan TCY. Astigmatism Correction Using SMILE. Asia Pac J Ophthalmol (Phila). 2019;8(5):391-6.

37. Dingeldein SA, and Klyce SD. The topography of normal corneas. Arch Ophthalmol. 1989;107:512-18.

38. Durr GM, Auvinet E, Ong JA, Gilca M, Choronzey ME, Meunier J. Enantiomorphism Of The Human Cornea Based On Corneal Topography 3D Atlas Analysis. IOVS. 2012;53:5569.

39. Febbraro JL, Koch DD, Khan HN, Saad A, Gatinel D. Detection of static cyclotorsion and compensation for dynamic cyclotorsion in laser in situ keratomileusis. J Cataract Refract Surg. 2010;36(10):1718-23.

40. Feng MT, Kim JT, Ambrósio R Jr, Belin MW, Grewal SPS, Yan W. International Values of Central Pachymetry in Normal Subjects by Rotating Scheimpflug Camera. Asia Pac J Ophthalmol (Phila). 2012;1(1):13-8.

41. Fernández J, Rodríguez-Vallejo M, Martínez J, Tauste A, Hueso E, Piñero DP. Confounding sizing in posterior chamber phakic lens selection due to white-to-white measurement bias. Indian J Ophthalmol. 2019;67(3):344-9.

42. Freedman KA, Brown SM, Mathews SM, Young RSL. Pupil size and the ablation zone in laser refractive surgery: considerations based on geometric optics. J Cataract Refract Surg. 2003;29: 1924-31.

43. Frost A, Ritter DJ, Trotter A, Pulia MS. Acute angle-closure glaucoma secondary to a phakic intraocular lens: an ophthalmic emergency. Clin Pract Cases Emerg Med. 2019;3(2):137-9.

44. Galletti JD, Ruiseñor Vázquez PR, Minguez N, Delrivo M, Bonthoux FF, Pförtner T. Corneal Asymmetry Analysis by Pentacam Scheimpflug Tomography for Keratoconus Diagnosis. J Refract Surg. 2015;31(2):116-23.

45. García-López V, García-López C, de Juan V, Martin R. Analysis of cataract surgery induced astigmatism: two polar methods comparison. J Optom. 2017;10(4):252-7.

46. Gharaee H, Shafiee M, Hoseini R, Abrishami M, Abrishami Y, Abrishami M. Angle Kappa Measurements: Normal Values in Healthy Iranian Population Obtained With the Orbscan II. Iran Red Crescent Med J. 2014;17(1):e17873. Published 2014 Dec 25. doi:10.5812/ircmj.17873.

47. Gomes JAP, Tan D, Rapuano CJ, Belin MW, Ambrósio Jr R, Guell JL, et al. Global Consensus on Keratoconus and Ectatic Disease. Cornea. 2015;34(4):359-69.

48. Greenstein SA1, Shah VP, Fry KL, Hersh PS. Corneal thickness changes after corneal collagen crosslinking for keratoconus and corneal ectasia: one-year results. J Cataract Refract Surg. 2011;37(4):691-700.

49. Haldipurkar SS, Shikari HT, Gokhale V. Wound construction in manual small incision cataract surgery. Indian J Ophthalmol. 2009;57(1):9-13.

50. Hall GW, Krischer C, Mobasher B, Rajan SD. The construction of sutureless cataract incision and the management of corneal astigmatism. Curr Opin Ophthalmol. 1993;4(1):33-8.

51. Hall JN. Inter-rater reliability of ward rating scales. Br J Psychiatry. 1974;125:248-55.

52. Hammond SD Jr, Puri AK, Ambati BK. Quality of vision and patient satisfaction after LASIK. Curr Opin Ophthalmol. 2004;15:328-32.

53. Hashemi H, Khabazkhoob M, Soroush S, Shariati R, Miraftab M, Yekta A. The location of incision in cataract surgery and its impact on induced astigmatism. Curr Opin Ophthalmol. 2016;27(1):58-64.

54. Haw W, Manche E. Effect of preoperative pupil measurements on glare, halos, and visual function after photoastigmatic refractive keratectomy. J Cataract Refract Surg. 2001;27:907-16.

55. Hayashi K, Ogawa S, Yoshida M, Yoshimura K. Wound stability and surgically induced corneal astigmatism after transconjunctival single-plane sclerocorneal incision cataract surgery. Jpn J Ophthalmol. 2017;61(1):113-23.

56. Hayashi K, Yoshida M, Hirata A, Yoshimura K. Changes in shape and astigmatism of total, anterior, and posterior cornea after long versus short clear corneal incision cataract surgery. J Cataract Refract Surg. 2018;44(1):39-49.

57. Hiep NX, Khanh PTM, Quyet D, Thai TV, Nga VT, Dinh TC, et al. Correcting Corneal Astigmatism with Corneal Arcuate Incisions during Femtosecond Laser Assisted Cataract Surgery. Open Access Maced J Med Sci. 2019;7(24):4260-5.

58. Ho JD, Liou SW, Tsai RJ, Tsai CY. Effects of aging on anterior and posterior corneal astigmatism. Cornea. 2010;29(6):632-7.

59. Ho JD, Tsai CY, Liou SW. Accuracy of corneal astigmatism estimation by neglecting the posterior corneal surface measurement. Am J Ophthalmol. 2009;147:788-95.

60. Hoffmann EM, Lamparter J, Mirshahi A, Elflein H, Hoehn R, Wolfram C, et al. Distribution of Central Corneal Thickness and its Association with Ocular Parameters in a Large Central European Cohort: The Gutenberg Health Study. PLoS One. 2013;8(8):e66158. doi:10.1371/journal.pone.0066158.

61. Holladay J. Holladay Report on the Pentacam. Pentacam HR® User Manual. Oculus, Wetzlar, Germany.

62. Holladay JT, Janes JA. Topographic changes in corneal asphericity and effective optical zone after laser in situ keratomileusis. J Cataract Refract Surg. 2002;28:942-7.

63. Holladay JT. Detecting Forme Fruste Keratoconus with the Pentacam. Supplement to Cataract & Refractive Surgery Today. 2008;11:12.

64. Holopainen JM1, Krootila K. Transient corneal thinning in eyes undergoing corneal cross-linking. Am J Ophthalmol. 2011;152(4):533-6.

65. Jiminez-Alfaro I, Benitez del Castillo JM, Garcia-Feijoo J, Gil de Bernabé JG, Serrano de La Iglesia JM. Safety of posterior chamber phakic intraocular lenses for the correction of high myopia: anterior segment changes after posterior chamber phakic intraocular lens implantation. Ophthalmology. 2001;108:90-9.

66. Jiminez-Alfaro I, Garcia-Feijoo J, Perez-Santonji JJ, Cuiña R. Ultrasound biomicroscopy of ZSAL-4 anterior chamber phakic intraocular lenses for high myopia. J Refract Surg. 2001;17:641-5.

67. Jinabhai A, Radhakrishnan H, O'Donnell C. Pellucid corneal marginal degeneration: a review. Cont Lens Ant Eye. 2011;34: 56-63.

68. Jones-Jordan LA, Walline JJ, Sinnott LT, Kymes SM, Zadnik K. Asymmetry in keratoconus and vision-related quality of life. Cornea. 2013;32(3):267-72.

69. Kanellopoulos AJ, Asimellis G. Revisiting keratoconus diagnosis and progression classification based on evaluation of corneal asymmetry indices, derived from Scheimpflug imaging in keratoconic and suspect cases. Clinical Ophthalmology. 2013;7:1539-48.

70. Kessel L, Andresen J, Tendal B, Erngaard D, Flesner P, Hjortdal J. Toric Intraocular Lenses in the Correction of Astigmatism During Cataract Surgery: A Systematic Review and Meta-analysis. Ophthalmology. 2016;123(2):275-86.

71. Khachikian SS, Belin MW, Ambrosio Jr R. Normative data for the oculus pentacam. In: Belin MW, Khachikian SS, Ambrosio Jr R (Eds). Elevation Based Corneal Tomography, 2nd edn. Jaypee-Highlights Medical Publisher, Inc.; 2012 .pp. 71-9.

72. Kiely PM, Carney LG, Smith G. Diurnal variations of corneal topography and thickness. Am J Optom Physiol Opt. 1982;59: 976-82.

73. Kiely PM, Smith G, Carney L.G. The mean shape of the human cornea. Optica Acta. 1982; 29(8):1027-40.

74. Kim G, Christiansen SM, Moshirfar M. Change in keratometry after myopic laser in situ keratomileusis and photorefractive keratectomy. J Cataract Refract Surg. 2014;40(4):564-74.

75. Kligman BE, Baartman BJ, Dupps WJ Jr. Errors in Treatment of Lower-order Aberrations and Induction of Higher-order Aberrations in Laser Refractive Surgery. Int Ophthalmol Clin. 2016;56(2):19-45.

76. Klyce SD. Chasing the suspect: keratoconus. Br J Ophthalmol. 2009;93:845-7.

77. Koch DD, Ali SF, Weikert MP, Shirayama M, Jenkins R, Wang L. Contribution of posterior corneal astigmatism to total corneal astigmatism. J Cataract Refract Surg. 2012;38(12):2080-7.

78. Koch DD, Jenkins RB, Weikert MP, Yeu E, Wang L. Correcting astigmatism with toric intraocular lenses: effect of posterior corneal astigmatism. J Cataract Refract Surg. 2013;39(12):1803-9.

79. Koch PS. Structural analysis of cataract incision construction. J Cataract Refract Surg. 1991;17 (Suppl):661-7.

80. Kodjikian L, Gain P, Donate D, Rouberol F, Burillon C. Malignant glaucoma induced by a phakic posterior chamber intraocular lens for myopia. J Cataract Refract Surg. 2002;28:2217-21.

81. Koller T1, Pajic B, Vinciguerra P, Seiler T. Flattening of the cornea after collagen crosslinking for keratoconus. J Cataract Refract Surg. 2011;37(8):1488-92.

82. Krachmer JH, Feder RS, Belin MW. Keratoconus and related noninflammatory corneal thinning disorders. Surv Ophthalmol. 1984;28:293-322.

83. Lazreg S, Mesplié N, Praud D, Delcourt C, Kamoun H, Chahbi M, et al. Comparison of corneal thickness and biomechanical properties between North African and French patients. J Cataract Refract Surg. 2013;39(3):425-30.

84. Lee BW, Jurkunas UV, Harissi-Dagner M, Poothullil AM, Tobaigy FM, Azar DT. Ectatic disorders associated with a claw-shaped pattern on corneal topography. Am J Ophthalmol. 2007;144(1):154 -6.

85. Lee H, Kang DSY, Choi JY, Ha BJ, Kim EK, Seo KY, et al. Analysis of pre-operative factors affecting range of optimal vaulting after implantation of 12.6-mm V4c implantable collamer lens in myopic eyes. BMC Ophthalmol. 2018;18(1):163.

86. Li X, Rabinowitz YS, Rasheed K, Yang H. Longitudinal study of the normal eyes in unilateral keratoconus patients. Ophthalmology. 2004;111(3):440-6.

87. Li X, Yang H, Rabinowitz YS. Keratoconus: classification scheme based on Videokeratography and clinical signs. J Cataract Refract Surg. 2009;35(9):1597-603.

88. Li Y, Shekhar R, Huang D. Corneal pachymetry mapping with high-speed optical coherence tomography. Ophthalmology. 2006;113(5):792-9.

89. Li Y, Tang M, Zhang X, Salaroli CH, Ramos JL, Huang D. Pachymetric mapping with Fourier domain optical coherence tomography. J Cataract Refract Surg. 2010;36(5):826-31.

90. Liang JL, Xing XL, Yang XT, Jiang YF, Zhang H. Clinical comparison analysis in surgically induced astigmatism of the total, anterior and posterior cornea after 2.2-mm versus 3.0-mm clear corneal incision cataract surgery. 2019;55(7):495-501.

91. Lim CW, Somani S, Chiu HH, Maini R, Tam ES. Astigmatic Outcomes of Single, Non-Paired Intrastromal Limbal Relaxing Incisions during Femtosecond Laser-Assisted Cataract Surgery Based on a Custom Nomogram. Clin Ophthalmol. 2020;14:1059-70.

92. Lim L, Wei RH, Chan WK, Tan DT. Evaluations of keratoconus in Asians: role of Orbscan II and Tomey TMS-2 corneal topography. Am J Ophthalmol. 2007;143:390-400.

93. Linke SJ, Baviera J, Munzer G, Fricke OH, Richard G, Katz T. Mesopic pupil size in a refractive surgery population (13,959 eyes). Optom Vis Sci. 2012;89(8):1156-64.

94. Litoff D, Belin MW, Winn SS. PAR Technology Corneal Topography System. Inv Ophthalmol Vis Sci. 1991;32:922.

95. Liu Q, Yang X, Lin L, Liu M, Lin H, Liu F, et al. Review on Centration, Astigmatic Axis Alignment, Pupil Size and Optical Zone in SMILE. Asia Pac J Ophthalmol (Phila). 2019;8(5):385-90.

96. Lovisolo CF, Reinstein DZ. Phakic intraocular lenses. Surv Ophthalmol. 2005;50:549-87.

97. Mahon L, Kent D. Can true monocular keratoconus occur? Clin Exp Optom. 2004;87:126.

98. Matsumoto Y, Hara T, Chiba K, Chikuda M. Optimal incision sites to obtain an astigmatism-free cornea after cataract surgery with a 3.2-mm sutureless incision. J Cataract Refract Surg. 2001;27(10):1615-9.

99. Miraftab M, Fotouhi A, Hashemi H, Jafari F, Shahnazi A, Asgari S. A modified risk assessment scoring system for post laser in situ keratomileusis ectasia in topographically normal patients. J Ophthalmic Vis Res. 2014;9(4):434-8.

100. Mohamed Mostafa E. Effect of Flat Cornea on Visual Outcome after LASIK. J Ophthalmol. 2015;2015:794854.

101. Monaco G, Scialdone A. Long-term outcomes of limbal relaxing incisions during cataract surgery: aberrometric analysis. Clin Ophthalmol. 2015;9:1581-7.

102. Moshirfar M, Edmonds JN, Behunin NL, Christiansen SM. Current options in the management of pellucid marginal degeneration. J Refract Surg. 2014;30(7):474-85.

103. Moshirfar M, Hoggan RN, Muthappan V. Angle Kappa and its importance in refractive surgery. Oman J Ophthalmol. 2013;6(3):151-8.

104. Muftuoglo O, Ayar O, Ozulken K, Ozyol E, Akıncı A. Posterior corneal elevation and back difference corneal elevation in diagnosing forme fruste keratoconus in the fellow eyes of unilateral keratoconus patients. J Cataract Refract Surg. 2013;39:1348-57.

105. Muftuoglu O, Alio JL. Anterior chamber angle-supported complications. In: Alió JL, Azar DT (Eds). Management of Complications in Refractive Surgery. Berlin: Springer-Verlag; 2008 .pp. 236.

106. Muftuoglu O, Ayar O, Hurmeric V, Orucoglu F , Kılıc I. Comparison of multimetric D index with keratometric, pachymetric, and posterior elevation parameters in diagnosing subclinical keratoconus in fellow eyes of asymmetric keratoconus patients. J Cataract Refract Surg. 2015;41:557-65.

107. Munnerlyn CR, Koons SJ, Marshall J. Photorefractive keratecomy: a technique for laser refractive surgery. J Refratc Surg. 1988;14:46-52.

108. Nilforoushan MR, Speaker M, Marmor M. Comparative evaluation of refractive surgery candidates with Placido topography, Orbscan II, Pentacam, and wavefront analysis. J Cataract Refract Surg. 2008;34:623-31.

109. Noor IH, Seiler TG, Noor K, Seiler T. Continued Long-term Flattening After Corneal Cross-linking for Keratoconus. J Refract Surg. 2018;34(8):567-70.

110. Ong HS, Farook M, Tan BBC, Williams GP, Santhiago MR, Mehta JS. Corneal Ectasia Risk and Percentage Tissue Altered in Myopic Patients Presenting for Refractive Surgery. Clin Ophthalmol. 2019;13:2003-15.

111. Packer M. Meta-analysis and review: effectiveness, safety, and central port design of the intraocular collamer lens. Clin Ophthalmol. 2016;10:1059-77.

112. Patel V, Muhtaseb M. Endothelial cell loss after pIOL implantation for high myopia. J Cataract Refract Surg. 2008;34:1424-5.

113. Pentacam HR® user manual. Oculus, Wetzlar, Germany.

114. Pineda R 2nd, Chauhan T. Phakic Intraocular Lenses and their Special Indications. J Ophthalmic Vis Res. 2016;11(4):422-8.

115. Pouliquen Y, Dhermy P, Espinasse MA, Savoldelli M. Keratoglobus. J Fr Ophthalmol. 1985;8(1):43-5.

116. Rabinowitz YS, Li X, Canedo ALC, Ambrósio Jr R, Bykhovskaya Y. Optical coherence tomography (OCT) combined with videokeratography to differentiate mild keratoconus subtypes. J Refract Surg. 2014;30(2):80-7.

117. Rabinowitz YS, McDonnell PJ. Computer-assisted corneal topography in keratoconus. Refract Corneal Surg. 1989;5:400-8.

118. Rabinowitz YS, Nesburn AB, McDonnell PJ. Videokeratography of the fellow eye in unilateral keratoconus. Ophthalmology. 1993;100:181-6.

119. Rabinowitz YS. Keratoconus. Surv Ophthalmol. 1998;42:297-319.

120. Rabinowitz YS. Videokeratographic indices to aid in screening for keratoconus. J Refract Surg. 1995;11(5):371-9.

121. Ramos IC, Correa R, Guerra FP, William Trattler, Michael W Belin, Stephen D Klyce, et al. Variability of subjective classifications of corneal maps from LASIK candidates. J Refract Surg. 2013;29(11):770-5.

122. Randleman JB, Woodward M, Lynn MJ, Stulting RD. Risk Assessment for Ectasia after Corneal Refractive Surgery. Ophthalmology. 2008;115:37-50.

123. Rasheed K, Rabinowitz YS, Remba D, Remba MJ. Interobserver and intraobserver reliability of a classification scheme for corneal topographic patterns. BJ Ophthalmol. 1998;82:1401-6.

124. Reinstein DZ, Archer TJ, Carp JI. The Surgeon's Guide to SMILE. Slack Inc.; 2018.

125. Reinstein DZ, Archer TJ, Gobbe M, Silverman RH, Coleman DJ. Epithelial thickness in the normal cornea: 3D display with VHF ultrasound. J Refract Surg. 2008;24:571-81.

126. Rho CR, Joo CK. Effects of steep meridian incision on corneal astigmatism in phacoemulsification cataract surgery. J Cataract Refract Surg. 2012;38(4):666-71.

127. Rigi M, Al-Mohtaseb Z, Weikert MP. Astigmatism Correction in Cataract Surgery: Toric Intraocular Lens Placement Versus Peripheral Corneal Relaxing Incisions. Int Ophthalmol Clin. 2016;56(3):39-47.

128. Robin JB, Schanzlin DJ, Verity SM, Barron BA, Arffa RC, Suarez E, et al. Peripheral corneal disorders. Surv Ophthalmol. 1986;31: 1-36.

129. Rocha KM, Soriano ES, Chamon W, Chalita MR, Nosé W. Spherical aberration and depth of focus in eyes implanted with aspheric and spherical intraocular lenses (A prospective randomized study). Ophthalmology. 2007;114:2050-4.

130. Romero-Jimenez M, Santodomingo-Rubido J, Wolffsohn JS. Keratoconus: a review. Cont Lens Ant Eye. 2010;33:157-66.

131. ROSS JV. Keratoconus posticus generalis. Am J Ophthalmol. 1950;33:801-3.

132. Saad A, Gatinel D. Evaluation of total and corneal wavefront high order aberrations for the detection of forme fruste keratoconus. Invest Ophthalmol Vis Sci. 2012;53:2978-92.

133. Saad A, Gatinel D. Topographic and tomographic properties of forme fruste keratoconus corneas. IOVS. 2010;51:5546-55.

134. Saad A, Guilbert E, Gatinel D. Corneal Enantiomorphism in Normal and Keratoconic Eyes. J Refract Surg. 2014;30(8):542-7.

135. Saad A, Lteif Y, Azan E, Gatinel D. Biomechanical properties of keratoconus suspect eyes. IOVS. 2010;51(6):2912-6.

136. Sanchez-Galeana CA, Zadok D, Montes M, Cortés MA, Chayet AS. Refractory intraocular pressure increase after phakic posterior chamber intraocular lens implantation. Am J Ophthalmol. 2002;134:121-3.

137. Santhiago MR, Giacomin NT, Smadja D, Bechara SJ. Ectasia risk factors in refractive surgery. Clin Ophthalmol. 2016;10:713-20.

138. Santhiago MR, Smadja D, Gomes B, Wilson SE, Mello G, Monteiro MLR, et al. Role of Percentage of Tissue Altered (PTA) as a risk factor in eyes with Normal preoperative topography that developed Ectasia after LASIK. Invest Ophthalmol Vis Sci. 2014;55(13):1548. doi: https://doi.org/.

139. Santhiago MR. Percent tissue altered and corneal ectasia. Curr Opin Ophthalmol. 2016;27(4):311-5. doi:10.1097/ICU.0000000000000276.

140. Schallhorn SC, Kaupp SE, Tanzer DJ, Tidwell J, Laurent J, Bourque LB. Pupil size and quality of vision after LASIK. Ophthalmology. 2003;110:1606-14.

141. Schlegel Z, Hoang-Xuan T, Gatinel D. Comparison of and correlation between anterior and posterior corneal elevation maps in normal eyes and keratoconus-suspect eyes. J Cataract Refract Surg. 2008;34:789-95.

142. Schweitzer C, Roberts CJ, Mahmoud AM, Colin J, Maurice-Tison S, Kerautret J. Screening of forme fruste keratoconus with the ocular response analyzer. Invest Ophthalmol Vis Sci. 2010;51:2403-10.

143. Seiler T, Quurke AW. Iatrogenic keratectasia after LASIK in a case of forme fruste keratoconus. J Cataract Refract Surg. 1998;24:1007-9.

144. Senthil S, Choudhari NS, Vaddavalli PK, Murthy S, Reddy JC, Garudadri CS. Etiology and Management of Raised Intraocular Pressure following Posterior Chamber Phakic Intraocular Lens Implantation in Myopic Eyes. PLoS One. 2017;12 (2):e0172929.

145. Seo KY, Yang H, Kim WK, Nam SM. Calculations of actual corneal astigmatism using total corneal refractive power before and after myopic keratorefractive surgery. PLoS One. 2017;12(4):e0175268.

146. Shirayama-Suzuki M, Amano S, Honda N, Usui T, Yamagami S, Oshika T. Longitudinal analysis of corneal topography in suspect keratoconus. Br J Ophthalmol. 2009;93:815-19.

147. Sinjab MM, Youssef LN. Pellucid-like keratoconus. Available on: www.ncbi.nlm.nih.gov/pmc/articles/PMC3752625.

148. Sinjab MM. "Astigmatic Dissociation". Corneal Tomography in Clinical Practice (Pentacam System): Basics and Clinical Interpretation, 4th edn. Jaypee-Highlights Medical Publisher, Inc.; 2020 (In press).

149. Sinjab MM. "Classifications and Patterns of Keratoconus and Keratectasia". In: Quick Guide to the Management of Keratoconus. Heidelberg, Germany: Springer; 2012 .pp. 13-57.

150. Sinjab MM. "Corneal Power Maps". Corneal Tomography in Clinical Practice (Pentacam System): Basics and Clinical Interpretation, 4th edn. Jaypee-Highlights Medical Publisher, Inc.; 2020 (In press).

151. Sinjab MM. "Corneal Thickness Maps and Profiles." Corneal Tomography in Clinical Practice (Pentacam System): Basics and Clinical Interpretation, 4th edn. Jaypee-Highlights Medical Publisher, Inc.; 2020 (In press).

152. Sinjab MM. "Elevation Maps." Corneal topography in clinical practice (Pentacam System): Basics and Clinical Interpretation, 2nd edn. Jaypee-Highlights Medical Publisher, Inc.; 2012 .pp. 39-50.

153. Sinjab MM. "Entities Misdiagnosed as Ectasia." Corneal Tomography in Clinical Practice (Pentacam System): Basics and Clinical Interpretation, 4th edn. Jaypee-Highlights Medical Publisher, Inc.; 2020 (In press).

154. Sinjab MM. "Factors of False Findings." Corneal Tomography in Clinical Practice (Pentacam System): Basics and Clinical Interpretation, 4th edn. Jaypee-Highlights Medical Publisher, Inc.; 2020 (In press).

155. Sinjab MM. "Patterns and Classifications in Ectatic Corneal Disorders." In: Sinjab MM and Cummings AB (Eds). Corneal Collagen Cross Linking. Springer International Publishing Switzerland; 2017.

156. Sinjab MM. "Progression Criteria." Corneal Tomography in Clinical Practice (Pentacam System): Basics and Clinical Interpretation, 4th edn. Jaypee-Highlights Medical Publisher, Inc.; 2020 (In press).

157. Sinjab MM. "The Practical Subjective IOL Selection." Corneal Tomography in Clinical Practice (Pentacam System): Basics and Clinical Interpretation, 4th edn. Jaypee-Highlights Medical Publisher, Inc.; 2020 (In press).

158. Sinjab MM. "The Practical Subjective Scoring System." Corneal Tomography in Clinical Practice (Pentacam System): Basics and Clinical Interpretation, 4th edn. Jaypee-Highlights Medical Publisher, Inc.; 2020 (In press).

159. Sinjab MM. "Tomographic Characteristics of Ectatic Corneal Diseases." Corneal Tomography in Clinical Practice (Pentacam System): Basics and Clinical Interpretation, 4th edn. Jaypee-Highlights Medical Publisher, Inc.; 2020 (In press).

160. Smadja D, Touboul D, Cohen A, Doveh E, Santhiago MR, Mello GR, et al. Detection of Subclinical Keratoconus Using an Automated Decision Tree Classification. Am J Ophthalmol. 2013;156:237-46.

161. Smolek MK, Klyce SD, Hovis JK. The universal standard scale: proposed improvements to the American National Standard Institute (ANSI) scale for corneal topography. Ophthalmology. 2002;109:361-9.

162. Szczotka LB, Rabinowitz YS, Yang H. Influence of contact lens wear on the corneal topography of keratoconus. CLAO J. 1996;22:270-3.

163. Tjon-Fo-Sang MJ, de Faber JT, Kingma C, Beekhuis WH. Cyclotorsion: a possible cause of residual astigmatism in refractive surgery. J Cataract Refract Surg. 2002;28(4):599-602.

164. Tummanapalli SS, Maseedupally V, Mandathara P, Rathi VM, Sangwan VS. Evaluation of corneal elevation and thickness indices in pellucid marginal degeneration and keratoconus. J Cataract Refract Surg. 2013;39:56-65.

165. Ueno Y, Hiraoka T, Beheregaray S, Miyazaki M, Ito M, Oshika T. Age-related changes in anterior, posterior, and total corneal astigmatism. J Refract Surg. 2014;30(3):192-7.

166. Ueno Y, Hiraoka T, Miyazaki M, Ito M, Oshika T. Corneal thickness profile and posterior corneal astigmatism in normal corneas. Ophthalmology. 2015;122:1072-8.

167. Verrey K. Keratoglobe aigu. Ophthalmologica. 1947;114:284-8.

168. Visser N, Nuijts RMMA, de Vries NE, Bauer NJV. Visual outcomes and patient satisfaction after cataract surgery with toric multifocal intraocular lens implantation. J Cataract Refract Surg. 2011;37:2034-42.

169. Walker RN, Khachikian SS, Belin MW. Scheimpflug imaging of pellucid marginal degeneration. Cornea. 2008;27(8):963-6.

170. Wallang BS, Das S. Keratoglobus. Eye. 2013;27(9):1004-12.

171. Waring GO, Rabinowitz YS, Sugar J, Damiano R. Nomenclature for keratoconus suspects. Refract Corneal Surg. 1993;9(3):219-22.

172. WaveLight GmbH. WaveLight® Allegro Oculyzer™ 1074 User Manual (English). Erlangen: WaveLight GmbH; 2001.

173. Whang WJ, Yoo YS, Joo CK. Corneal power changes with Scheimpflug rotating camera after hyperopic LASIK. Medicine (Baltimore). 2018;97(50):e13306. doi:10.1097/MD.0000000000013306

174. Williams GS, Muhtaseb M. Safety Considerations for Phakic IOLs. CRSTEurope; 2012.

175. Wilson SE, Klyce SD, Husseini ZM. Standardized color-coded maps for corneal topography. Ophthalmology. 1993;100:1723-7.

176. Zadnik K, Steger-May K, Fink BA, Joslin CE, Nichols JJ, Rosenstiel CE, et al. CLEK Study Group. Between-eye asymmetry in keratoconus. Cornea. 2002;21(7):671-9.

177. Zhou J, Xu Y, Li M, Knorz MC, Zhou X. Preoperative refraction, age and optical zone as predictors of optical and visual quality after advanced surface ablation in patients with high myopia: a cross-sectional study. BMJ Open. 2018;8(6):e023877.

178. Zhu Y, Zhu H, Jia Y, Zhou J. Changes in anterior chamber volume after implantation of posterior chamber phakic intraocular lens in high myopia. BMC Ophthalmol. 2018;18(1):185.

Other Cited Material

A. Michelson MA, Myers RA. Corneal higher order aberrations and visual dysfunction with multifocal IOLs. Paper presented at: American Society of Cataract & Refractive Surgery Annual Meeting. Chicago; April 20-24, 2012.

B. Hamza I, Aly MG, Hashem KA, "Multifocal IOL Dissatisfaction in Patients with High Coma Aberrations," presented at the ASCRS Symposium on Cataract, IOL and Refractive Surgery, San Diego, California, USA; March 2011.

Index

Page numbers followed by *f* refer to figure, and *t* refer to table.